THE
BIGGEST
SECRET
IN
WOMEN'S
HEALTH

Stigma, Indifference, Outrage, and Optimism

SHERRIE PALM

Foreword by Marco Pelosi III, MD

P⬤P

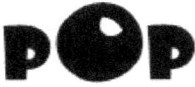

POP Publishing and Distribution

Hardcover: ISBN # 978-0-9855356-5-0
Softcover: ISBN # 978-0-9855356-4-3
Kindle: ISBN # 978-0-9855356-6-7

POP Illustrations by Love & Logic

Edited by Joyline 'Jo' Maenzanise

MEDICAL DISCLAIMER

Every human being born with a vagina has been handed their first risk of experiencing pelvic organ prolapse. Pregnancy elicits the second risk, typically closely followed by the third risk, childbirth. In those who live long enough to experience menopause, the fourth risk often brings to the front-page symptoms that may have been hovering subliminally for the right set of circumstances to reveal health concerns rarely talked about openly or comfortably in the past. The intent of this book is to increase awareness of pelvic organ prolapse ahead of the curve rather than following diagnosis.

The material provided in this book is meant for informational and educational use only. It is not intended to replace guidance or care from health care practitioners. If you believe you have symptoms of pelvic organ prolapse (POP) or any other illness, consult with the appropriate healthcare professional for diagnosis and treatment. If the insights you receive from your healthcare provider do not satisfy your needs, seek advice from additional healthcare professionals. Neither the author nor the publisher is liable for the misuse or misinterpretation of information provided in this book.

With love to Great Uncle Norm, for being a subliminal source of female empowerment.

"You come from a long line of strong women."

"When vaginal and intimate health are given the same respect as women's heart, hormone, and breast health, women will finally capture health equity."

Sherrie Palm

TESTIMONIALS

"The general public still lives in darkness. I have seen this in my 30+ year career as a urogynecologist. So now I have a friend who brings light to this issue of POP and is a champion for women worldwide. Without her advocate role, many women would continue to suffer in silence physically and emotionally. Sherrie's goal in her professional life is to educate and bring to the front the hope of relief, the hope of care, the hope of cure. We need Sherrie to teach us and help us understand how to address women's needs to hold back this silent epidemic."

Red Alinsod, MD, FACOG, FACS, ACGE
Cosmetic Urogynecologist
Alinsod Institute for Aesthetic Vulvovaginal Surgery

"Sherrie Palm is an extraordinary advocate for women who are navigating POP. She has spent years conversing with and learning from both women with POP and clinicians who treat the condition. This book is a collaboration of that information. The reader is treated to a detailed road map of how to navigate POP. Every chapter begins with a patient quote. That patient voice throughout this book offers women hope, a sense of community, and validation. With each chapter, the reader will gain knowledge and become empowered. This book is a must-read for all women and those who love them.

When Sherrie was diagnosed and treated for POP, she not only

*recognized that we women did not have information, she also rec-
ognized that we did not have community. Her initiative to found
the APOPS advocacy nonprofit and to write books addressing POP
has changed lives and continues to change lives every day. Her resolve
to obliterate the stigma attached to POP and POP symptoms is
palpable throughout her work as she speaks about POP as just another health condition. Sherrie is such an inspiration as she continues
her crusade to educate women, healthcare providers, and academics
about the impact POP has on lives.*

*Thank you, Sherrie Palm, for modeling passion, compassion, tenac-
ity, and persistence and for encouraging and empowering women to
use their voices because it is true - every voice matters."*

Mary Pippen
Patient, Kentucky/USA

*"Sherrie Palm is an army trapped in a woman's body and that army
is ignited. She is the passionate and tireless voice for the intimate
problems that afflict over 50 million women. She wields amazing
influence within the medical community, the medical industry, and
patient groups. I know. I've witnessed it."*

Marco Pelosi III MD, FACOG, FACS, FICS, FAACS
Cosmetic Gynecologist, Founder
Int'l Society of Cosmetic Gynecologists

*"Sher Palm carries the torch. Throughout my 45-year career in the
nonprofit sector, I have worked with countless individuals and organizations championing causes that transform the quality of life
in our communities and our world, their passion often the result
of their own lived experiences, i.e., homelessness, addiction, child
abuse, hunger, breast cancer, mental illness. Sher Palm stands out as
a fierce advocate and champion. Her journey with her own pelvic
organ prolapse diagnosis fueled her passion to commit her whole
being to APOPS, advancing and leading a never before vaginal and
intimate health evolution. Sitting at the table alongside patients,*

healthcare, academia, researchers, policymakers, and advocates, she inspires, she leads, she is the bridge that unites all sectors that are part and parcel of progression in the POP space."

Susanne Vella ~ Nonprofit Professional
Former APOPS Board Director

"APOPS, with Sherrie Palm leading the organization, has been at the forefront of educating and assisting women with pelvic organ prolapse (POP). This new book will continue the good work being done by APOPS and will provide women with essential and timely information on POP where there continues to be a lack of awareness and care for women with this condition."

Elizabeth LaGro, MLIS, Vice President
The Simon Foundation for Continence

"I have never met a person as dedicated to pelvic health awareness as Sherrie Palm. Sherrie's commitment to de-stigmatizing sexual and pelvic health has created a strong current that is now being felt around the world. The wave of change is coming, and its strongest voice is Sherrie Palm."

Suny Caminero, MD
Aesthetic Gynecologist
Cosmetic Gynecology Florida

ACKNOWLEDGEMENTS

CONTRIBUTORS

My heartfelt gratitude to the patients and women's pelvic health medical practitioners who contributed to this book and share POP knowledge and experiences daily to cultivate pelvic organ prolapse awareness and understanding.

PRACTITIONERS

Note: Both gynecologists and urologists may subspecialize as Female Pelvic Medicine Reconstructive Surgeons (FPMRS). At the time of book publication, a discussion was stirring within the practitioner governing bodies American Board of Obstetrics and Gynecology (ABOG), the American Board of Urology (ABU), and the American Board of Medical Specialties (ABMS), considering a name change to clarify accreditation. For ease of understanding, the term urogynecologist will be used in this book to reference both gynecologists and urologists who are Female Pelvic Medicine Reconstructive Surgeons.

Red Alinsod, MD/USA, *Cosmetic Urogynecologist*
Hichem Bensmail, MD/France, *Cosmetic Urogynecologist*
Claudio Catalisano, MD/Italy, *Cosmetic Gynecologist*
Hugo H Davila, MD/USA, *FPMRS Urologist*
John De Lancey, MD/USA, FPMRS *Urogynecologist*
Roger Dmochowski, MD/USA, *FPMRS Urologist*
Fulya Dökmeci, MD, Professor/Turkey, *Urogynecologist*
Alexandra Dubinskaya, MD/USA, *FPMRS Urogynecologist*
Carlos Errando-Smet, PhD, MD/Spain, *FPMRS Urologist*
Enrico Finazzi Agro, MD/Italy, *FPMRS Urologist*
Michael Goodman, MD/USA, *Cosmetic Gynecologist*

Cheryl Iglesia, MD/USA, *Urogynecologist*
Stephanie Molden, *MD/USA, Cosmetic Urogynecologist*
Ana Belén Muñoz Menéndez, *MD/Spain, Urogynecologist*
Debra Muth, ND/USA, NP, APRN Naturopath
Charles Nager, MD/USA, *Urogynecologist*
Hedwig Neels, PT, Ph.D./Amsterdam, *Physical Therapist*
Barry O'Reilly, MD/Ireland, *Urogynecologist*
Marco Pelosi III, MD/USA, *Cosmetic Gynecologist*
Inés Ramírez, PT, Ph.D./Spain, *Physical Therapist*
Michael Reed, MD/USA, *Cosmetic Gynecologist*
Jan-Paul Roovers, MD/ Netherlands, *Urogynecologist*
Barbara Settles-Huge, PT/USA *Physical Therapist*
Beth Shelly, DPT /USA, *Physical Therapist*
Abbas Shobieri, MD/USA, *Urogynecologist*
Andrew Siegel, MD/USA, *FPMRS Urologist*
Adrian Wagg, MD/Canada, *FRCP Geriatrician*

Thank you to the practitioners who opted out of sharing insights due to conflict of interest; your honesty and integrity speaks for itself.

PATIENTS AND PERSONAL

Advancing social norms is no easy task, especially when related to stigmatized vaginal and sexual health concerns. My eternal gratitude to:

- The enlightened and empowered POP*Stars, women within the APOPS patient support community who recognize APOPS vision significance and share deeply personal experiences with each other to advance women's health.

- Gram, my guiding light and most impactful source of love and inspiration.

- My son Erik for his continual and unconditional support.

- My father who taught me the value of humor and tenacity.

- The DBC for the whispers of guidance they provide.

- M and M.

- Norma and Gordy.

- Mary Pippen, my soul sister, whose compassionate heart lifts me up.

- Maripat Francis Voellmecke for initial editing assistance.

- APOPS' dedicated Forum Administrative Team who generously volunteer time to keep the ship running smoothly behind the curtain.

  Larissa Bossaer
  Stephanie Cerniglia
  Cindy Heidel
  Eileen Healy McQuiggan
  Nicole Moorley
  Mary Pippen
  Whitney Smith
  Kathy Vater

- APOPS Board of Directors for their vision.

  Sherrie Palm, APOPS Founder
  Mary Pippen
  Melissa Frasure
  Michele Modellas
  Alesa Arnett
  Gina Vorhees

PRO-BONO SERVICES

With warm appreciation to the generous individuals and companies who have shared treatment insights, pro-bono services, and product donations to propel APOPS efforts.

Holistic & Transitional Healing Insights
Debra Muth, ND, WHNP, APNP, BAAHP Founder
Serenity Health Care Center
www.serenityhealthcarecenter.com

Spanish Translations
Ana Belén Muñoz Menéndez, Urogynaecologist, MD, PhD
Marqués de Valdecilla University Hospital
www.twitter.com/uspvaldecilla

Medical Device & Wearable Donations

Leva
Axena Health
www.axenahealth.com/

Perifit
www.perifit.co

Squeezy App
www.squeezyapp.com

SRC Health
www.srchealth.com

POP Imagery and Design Services
Angela Roche
Love & Logic
www.loveandlogic.co.uk

Branded Merchandise Donations
James Warner & Kathy Walker
First Impressions Promotion
www.firstimpressionspromotions.com

Accounting & Services
Andrew Holman, CPA

Dave Chesson Kindlepreneur
www.kindlepreneur.com

Legal Counsel & Services
Marquette Nonprofit Clinic, Marquette Law School
www.marquettelegalclinic.org

Heartfelt appreciation to the individuals who provided services to APOPS and prefer to remain anonymous.

FOREWORD

Marco A. Pelosi III, MD

Rare would be the individual with the drive, the passion, and the ability to forge a movement in the medical world from the ground up. Rarer still if such a person was neither a healthcare professional nor a scientist. Yet the work in your hands is the product of the engaging force of a very real and present mover and shaker.

Her name is Sherrie Palm. Over a decade ago, she was a patient with prolapse. Today, she's the world's leading patient advocate for prolapse, well-known to physicians and afflicted women worldwide. What has fueled her fire from the beginning is the huge educational chasm that exists among physicians and affected women in every country. Top on her bucket list is to have prolapse screening much more accessible than it is today so that preventive measures can be instituted in the early stages.

I am a gynecologic pelvic surgeon trained in both prolapse repairs and aesthetics. I also run a society devoted to the same. A few years ago, I started a Facebook discussion group and a podcast to expand society's reach. While mining and recruiting talent for these pursuits online, Sherrie Palm showed up on my LinkedIn radar screen. From our first conversation, it was obvious that she, the society, the discussion groups, and I shared many of the same goals. She invited me to join her prolapse patient group simply to listen to the stories of real women with real problems straight from the source. The rest is history.

Pelvic organ prolapse is not just another medical condition. It is the most common lifestyle-altering female medical condition in the world. It exists on a spectrum of severity and afflicts over half of all mothers globally. The numbers are staggering yet rarely mentioned. For many, simple lifestyle modifications are available to improve their quality of life. For others, a variety of management options exist, and many are in development. Curiously, public awareness of prolapse is even low among many clinicians, despite the ease and economy with which it can be assessed.

What Sherrie Palm has accomplished in this work is unique in the field of pelvic organ prolapse. She has combined the medical perspectives of a diverse group of innovative healthcare professionals and the patient perspective representative of the thousands of women who have shared their day-to-day experiences living with prolapse. For healthcare professionals, it gives the real patient perspectives that far exceed anything ever found in the medical literature. Symptoms absent from clinical research are brought into view. For patients, this is the ultimate educational primer. It addresses their problems with expert commentary on state-of-the-art and a glimpse of the future.

Beginning with an exhaustive analysis of events that injure the pelvic floor, followed by the anatomical results of that damage, and then an equally immersive discussion of the symptoms caused by these injuries, the organization of the material is first-rate. Experts will gain useful insights from the symptomatology sections as they have been sourced to a large degree from Palm's large patient-only discussion groups. This foundational knowledge prepares the reader for detailed discussions of screening and management options that include traditional as well as new and promising techniques and technologies. The work moves on to provide a guided primer for patients to get the most out of their interactions with healthcare professionals.

This work cannot be any timelier. We live in an era of unprecedented access to information, yet crucial knowledge gets lost in a sea of noise. Since anyone can publish anything anytime without restriction, a filter to sift out the bad information, misinformation, and outdated information is immensely valuable to those who lack training, education, and experience in the field. Since patients find themselves increasingly rushed through a healthcare system that leaves less and less time for face-to-face discussion, a lens through which to view their concerns in robust detail is invaluable. Here, in a single resource, Palm presents both a filter and a lens of the highest quality. Through her years of passionate and driven research, she has done the heavy lifting of identifying an excellent representation of world experts and the women they serve. Bravo!

Marco A. Pelosi, III, MD, FACOG, FACS, FICS, FAACS
Cosmetic Gynecologist, Pelvic Surgeon, Aesthetic Surgeon
Founder, International Society of Cosmetic Gynecologists

THE VAGINA: THE MOST STIGMATIZED HEALTH FRONTIER

The subliminal message most women receive from early childhood is that the vagina and vulva are private, personal, best kept undercover, creating an atmosphere of stigma. By definition, stigma is a mark of disgrace associated with a particular circumstance or quality. It's no wonder women have such a difficult time decoding vaginal health.

Women are rarely familiar with pelvic organ prolapse (POP) prior to the pivotal examination clarifying the condition has manifested. Discovery upon diagnosis is unfortunately often the end result of months, sometimes years, experiencing painful, awkward, or embarrassing POP symptoms. Physically incapacitating to varying degrees based on type(s) and grades of severity, POP makes a mess out of nearly every aspect of women's lives. POP stigma often generates feelings of shame, distress, helplessness, anxiety, blame, hopelessness, isolation, embarrassment, and fear. Frequently the stigma overlaps with shock given the cryptic nature of POP.

> "The Biggest Secret shines a light into the dark recesses of female anatomy, and lifts the taboo surrounding female vaginal health. It openly explains the remarkably common problems that women with prolapse suffer so they are no longer isolated in their experiences. This book also delivers essential information for women so they can understand mysterious changes going on within their bodies."
> ~John De Lancey, MD

I was absolutely stunned to be diagnosed with POP; there was not even a whisper on my health radar despite pandemic prevalence. I found it unnerving to be told I had a condition that is quite common and yet I was clueless existed. I'd done "the right stuff" regarding routine women's wellness checks including pelvic exams, mammograms, and hormone supplementation.

I attributed symptoms that began manifesting in my late 30's to be part of the normal aging process. I obviously recognized that tissues bulging out of my vaginal canal in my 50's had to indicate something relatively significant. However, prior to that unsettling symptom, loss of Kegel contraction strength, inability to keep a tampon in, difficulty starting my urine stream, abdominal bloat, and chronic constipation were all symptoms I had been experiencing. If I'd recognized they meant something significant enough to be addressed by a clinician rather than part of the aging process, would they have led me to an earlier diagnosis?

In the course of scouting for answers to address my needs, exasperation made me more and more determined to share the information I was uncovering with other women to encourage them to become informed about POP prior to diagnosis. This did not seem like one of those women's health issues that should be arbitrarily known. This seemed like a health issue that all women should be informed of ahead of the curve.

I asked multiple clinicians whose paths I crossed during my journey from diagnosis through treatment why I'd never heard of POP. I wanted to know why the topic had never come up during routine pelvic exams given the significant prevalence I was reading about online. I continually received the same response to my question: *women won't talk about it*. I found this both unsettling and unacceptable. Women need to be informed and educated about the significance of Kegels and PC muscle strength for general pelvic floor health, post-childbirth health, sexual health, and continence health. This enables women, whether young or mature, to recognize commonly occurring symptoms that are markers of POP.

At this point in women's health evolution, it is irrational that a common condition exists with little awareness. We must arouse open discussion to help women recognize POP symptoms. We must encourage vaginal dialogue to eradicate the associated health stigma. And we must also encourage patient/practitioner conversations about POP to advance this most notable facet of women's wellness.

Considering many women do not disclose or discuss embarrassing POP symptoms to their physicians, and POP screening seldom efficiently or effectively occurs prior to women noticing vaginal tissue bulge, it is not surprising that precise POP prevalence data is nonexistent. While estimated POP statistics are staggering, the reality is until screening is standardized and included in routine pelvic examinations, accurate prevalence data will fall short. Currently, many research and academic papers estimate that up to 50% of the female population will experience POP, or 50% of women who have given birth have POP, or 50% of menopausal women endure POP. According to the Wu study, the number of women with at least one pelvic floor disorder will increase from 28.1 million in 2010 to between 43.8 and 58.2 million in 2050. These figures are inclusive of breakdowns of an increase in the prevalence of urinary incontinence by 55%, fecal incontinence by 59%, and pelvic organ prolapse by 46%.

As acknowledgement of POP goes mainstream and global wellness initiatives shift, women will take comfort in the knowledge that they are not alone. Currently, women shy away from disclosing signs and symptoms of POP to others because of the stigma attached to tissues bulging out of the vagina, urinary or fecal incontinence, and sexual dysfunction. Broad-spectrum POP awareness and public dissemination are key to reducing stigma and generating an open, comfortable mindset regarding vaginal health, the most guarded aspect of women's wellness.

Along my journey, I have been incredibly fortunate to meet many progressive healthcare stakeholders and policymakers who recognize the transformation coming into women's health. I am also very privileged to communicate with women mid-teens through the end of life from around the world who ask every single day why they were neither informed of nor screened for POP ahead of the curve.

POP is a global pandemic health concern. It is appalling that it remains a cloaked hurdle in women's wellness. It is imperative healthcare, academia, research, industry, and policy work side by side to stimulate the next evolution of and revolution in women's health.

POP is one of the most significant challenges women will address in the on-going battle to attain health ballast for our gender. I encourage all women to take control of their pelvic health and to recognize that they have the capacity to find the answers they seek. For a female health condition to be shrouded in silence because of embarrassment at this point in history, after all we have achieved as women, is unacceptable. As we push forward to increase POP awareness for the betterment of women's collective health, women will become familiar with this common, cryptic health concern, recognize symptoms, and seek appropriate medical intervention.

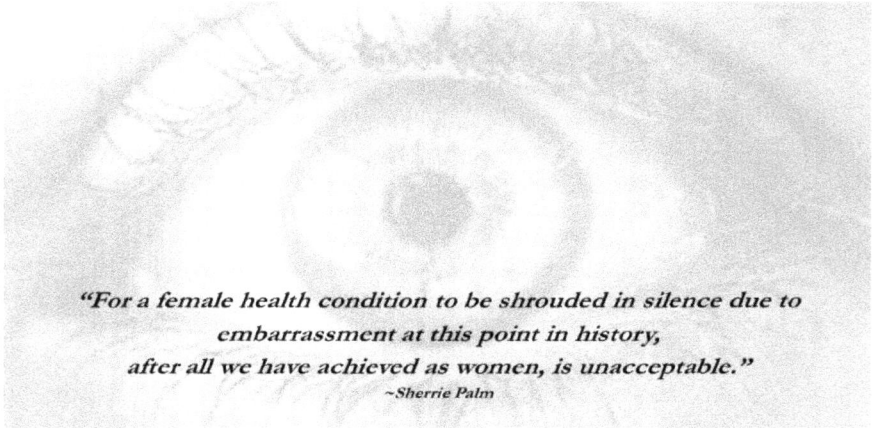

"For a female health condition to be shrouded in silence due to embarrassment at this point in history, after all we have achieved as women, is unacceptable."
~Sherrie Palm

Life lessons that cause the greatest pain, whether physical or emotional, remain firmly embedded in our subconscious. Devastated by what is occurring in their bodies, women experiencing POP can become empowered and recapture control once given the information and guidance needed to find their unique and individual health stability.

Women must speak out loudly and unabashedly about this last forbidden health frontier. As we continue to advance POP directives, increase awareness, and define needs, we will spawn a new era in women's health. And as we enable support and guidance, clarify misconceptions, and share insights within all sectors, we spearhead the evolution of POP treatment. The vagina is after all, both a vessel of life and love.

CONTENTS

TESTS AND TREATMENTS: ANALYZING THE OPTIONS

WHAT IS HAPPENING TO MY BODY?

1

PELVIC ORGAN PROLAPSE: THE BASICS

APOPS Patient Perspective: *"Women often enter the APOPS support forum feeling alone, powerless, and confused by their prolapse diagnosis. As they engage in the APOPS community, they are embraced and validated. By sharing their stories, women become strong, knowledgeable, confident, and empowered! Priceless!*
~MP, Kentucky/USA

In this time of enlightened self-help, it is hard to imagine a health condition that is highly prevalent yet mostly unacknowledged. POP is a women's health disorder that has been medically documented for nearly 4,000 years. It causes significant physical, emotional, social, sexual, fitness, and/or employment quality-of-life (QOL) impacts. Despite diverse paths of treatment, the majority of women have no knowledge it exists prior to diagnosis. Today's women are educated, self-reliant, pro-active. We seek answers to health dilemmas rather than brush them aside. When a health issue of any nature arises, we immediately hit Dr. Google and search for insights. So how is it possible POP has slipped past our radar?

Being told at the age of 54 that I was experiencing POP was a shock. My concern about the need to address this "new" health issue didn't upset me; that was obvious based on my symptoms, particularly the walnut-sized lump bulging out of my vagina. Discovering that I had a common condition that *I'd never heard of* - the progression of which I possibly could have reduced severity of with routine maintenance had I known about it earlier - infuriated me.

We have come a long way over the past 50 years regarding comfort with openly discussing health conditions related to our sexual anatomy. We comfortably acknowledge erectile dysfunction (ED), a personal and potentially embarrassing condition in which erection of the penis is difficult or impossible to achieve. Despite the stigma attached to the breast health campaign in its infancy, the indignity has all but disappeared. Yet there remains a significant shortfall in meaningful discussion about or reference to POP. Vaginal health is, without a doubt, the most stigmatized health frontier.

Many of the factors that contribute to POP occurrence were as prevalent in the days of early man as they are now. POP documentation dates back to the Kahun Gynaecologic Papyrus of Egyptian times, circa 1835 B.C.E. The word prolapse is Latin in origin, meaning "to fall". Hippocrates wrote about inserting a pomegranate into the vagina as a treatment for prolapse. Some women were subjected to succussion. This medical treatment consisted of tying the body upside down by the feet to a fixed ladder-like frame and repeatedly bouncing up and down until the prolapse was reduced. The women were then bed-bound for three days with their legs tied together (now there's a cocktail party conversation starter).

> *"Prolapse comes from the Latin word prolapsus ("a slipping forth"); this refers to a falling, slipping or downward displacement of an organ. Pelvic organ prolapse is thus, primarily, a definition of anatomical changes associated with symptoms. As a physician, we listen to our patients' symptoms to make the appropriate diagnosis, but POP is often a "silent" condition impacting quality of life. To overcome this barrier, we need to listen carefully and respectfully to identify POP and help our patients. Always, always listen to learn."*
>
> Hugo H Davila, MD

In general, POP in its entirety is not openly discussed. This silent pandemic needs to be openly and comfortably deliberated to enable women suffering in embarrassed silence with symptoms they don't understand to access diagnosis and treatment. The significance of pelvic floor anatomy should be emphasized to young women during high school fitness classes. Discussions during routine pelvic exams should include questions about POP symptoms to explore potential issues. Childbirth is the leading cause of POP, yet conversations rarely make it into classes. If we adjusted a few of the standardized processes in women's wellness protocol, recognition of pelvic floor issues and the reason for pelvic health maintenance would become common knowledge. As POP consciousness goes mainstream, the most beneficial awareness and navigational tools will become clear.

POP is a highly variable condition consisting of five types and four grades of severity. An organ or organs including the uterus, bladder, vagina, urethra, rectum, and/or intestines become displaced. The uterus can shift downward into and eventually push out of the vaginal canal. The balance of organs sit behind the vaginal wall tissue, but the organ bulge behind the vaginal wall protrudes into or outside of the vagina. Multiple types of POP can occur simultaneously.

The complex support structure within a woman's pelvic cavity includes ligaments, muscles, fascia, and soft connective tissues. These tissues support the organs from above and below to maintain their positions within the pelvic cavity. The two most important structures that provide support for pelvic organs are ligaments from above and the pubococcygeus muscle (PC) or pelvic floor muscle below. The PC muscle is a bowl-shaped trampoline-like band of muscle sitting at the base of the pelvic cavity. When any part of the pelvic organ support system is torn, damaged, or weakened, the structural integrity of the entire system is reduced, enabling organs to drop. Displaced pelvic organs can cause a wide variety of symptoms. POP generally worsens over time. Treatment is essential to restore quality of life.

Women's bodies are as unique on the inside as they are on the outside. This individuality makes it difficult to wrap a single set of boundaries around treatment options, which include surgical and nonsurgical choices. Undoubtedly POP is one of the most unsettling health concerns women address in their ongoing efforts to maintain health throughout their life cycle. As POP awareness accelerates, the field will continue to evolve, and the most beneficial tools will become evident.

The commonality of multiple aspects of female pelvic health is unsettling. However, accurate data for POP and related pelvic floor disorders is sorely lacking. Precise statistics for POP prevalence are impossible to validate globally due to a lack of standardized screening protocol, patient embarrassment blocking open dialogue, and insufficient POP curriculum provided in fields of medical practice providing pelvic examinations.

Statistics vary radically by study. The Mathias 2020 study of pelvic floor disorders focused on elderly women treated by primary health care. The sample size of 399 patients treated was extracted from a population of 16,905 women 60 years of age and older. It revealed that 70.2% of the women had at least one pelvic floor disorder. It additionally highlighted that while 77.5% of them had significant POP, only 22% of them reported symptoms. Clearly, stigma inhibits women from reporting these life-altering issues. Some eye-opening details from other studies indicate:

- The prevalence of POP differs by study from 3%-93% of women; 50% prevalence is a commonly quoted incidence.

- It is common for women to have more than one pelvic floor disorder.

- Women in mid-teens through end-of-life experience POP.

- There are more than 300,000 surgeries for POP annually in the US.

- Childbearing and menopause are the leading causes of POP, but multiple lifestyle, behavioral, and co-existing conditions increase risk of POP in women of all ages.

- Up to 40% of women experience sphincter damage during childbirth.

- 30% of women will undergo repeat surgery for POP.

- The number of women who will undergo surgery for POP is predicted to increase by 46% by 2050.

- In 2001, the estimated annual cost of surgical treatment for pelvic organ prolapse in the US surpassed $1 billion.

While pelvic organ prolapse is seldom life-threatening, it is nearly always life-altering. POP ultimately causes considerable distress, impacting multiple facets of a woman's lives. When you don't feel well, it is difficult to participate enthusiastically in any activity. When health concerns impact the capacity to care for your family, it prompts an emotional burden. Continuing to generate income becomes a serious challenge when physically uncomfortable or in pain on the job. At times, POP can also cause significant difficulty fulfilling employment responsibilities; this causes conflict in the workplace.

POP quality of life impacts do not discriminate by age, race, nationality, ethnicity, socio-economic dynamic, or socio-cultural status. It is unfortunate many women live their lives enduring symptoms they don't understand.

2

TYPES OF PELVIC ORGAN PROLAPSE

APOPS Patient Perspective: "*APOPS taught me that having POP is a journey, a process that includes anxiety, frustration, anger, and disbelief, which turns into acceptance and empowerment to make surgical or nonsurgical medical decisions suited specifically to fit my unique needs.*"

~DA, Oklahoma/USA

POP can simultaneously occur with more than one of the five types. Since the organs and tissues in the pelvic cavity are tightly grouped, and the functions of these organs, organ systems, and tissues are interrelated, it makes sense that women may experience diverse symptoms of POP. It is important that the practitioner you choose to treat POP is thorough and takes each kind of prolapse into consideration when guiding treatment. A POP subspecialist such as a urogynecologist or a physical therapist specializing in women's health is the most logical choice.

POP does not occur because of a defect in pelvic organs; it occurs because there is a weakness in or damage to the organ support structures. There are five types of POP.

- Cystocele

- Rectocele

- Uterine

- Vaginal Vault

- Enterocele

"POP appears in very different ways, and each woman feels it differently. It is possible that part of the vagina comes down (front, rear or top of the vagina), or it can be two or the three parts at the same time. The symptoms range from a feeling of heaviness in certain situations (especially when we make have abdominal pressure), to noticing a ball of tissue coming outside of the vagina or including other problems such as constipation or voiding difficulty. Some women don't care at all about the prolapse and some of them are so uncomfortable they need to treat it."

Ana Belén Muñoz Menéndez, MD

Cystocele

A cystocele occurs when the bladder bulges into the front vaginal wall. It pushes down toward the opening to the vagina and eventually through the vaginal opening to the outside of the body. The bladder and urethra prolapse together. (The urethra transports urine that's stored in the bladder out of the body as we urinate.) Cystocele symptoms are a frequent or urgent need to urinate in grades 1 or 2 of severity; this is considered early stage. Involuntary urinary leakage may include stress incontinence. This is leakage of urine during physical activities that increase intra-abdominal pressure such as coughing, sneezing, laughing, hard foot strike fitness activities, or sexual activity (referred to as coital incontinence). Urge urinary incontinence is a sudden, intense urge to urinate followed by an involuntary loss of urine. Overactive bladder is a frequent and sudden urge to urinate that may be difficult to control. Any of or a mixture of all three of these bladder issues is possible with cystocele. In the advanced grades of cystocele, it becomes difficult to start the urine stream. Incomplete emptying of the bladder may result, and the potential for urinary tract infections (UTI) increases.

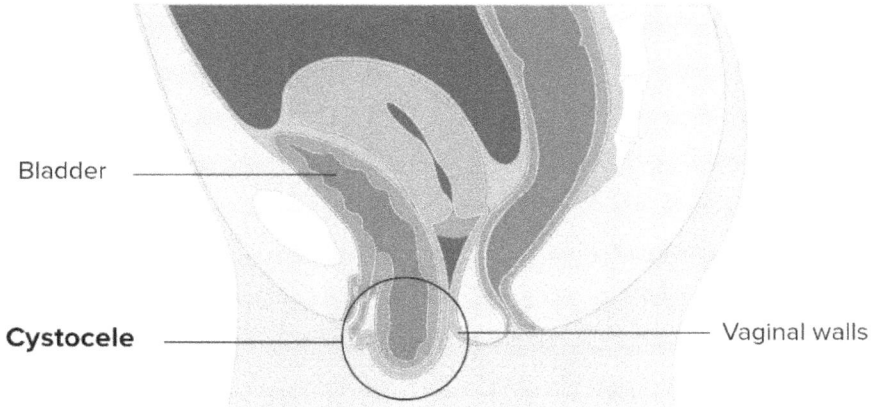

Cystocele. Image courtesy of Association for Pelvic Organ Prolapse Support.

Rectocele

A rectocele is a hernia bulge in the large bowel (rectum) pushes into the rear vaginal wall. Stool typically gets trapped in the hernia bulge, resulting in chronic constipation. Along with constipation, hemorrhoids, incomplete stool emptying, rectal pressure, bloating from gas buildup, general pelvic discomfort, or impacted stool may occur. Splinting (inserting one or two fingers into the vagina to push the hernia bulge back into place) may be necessary to enable bowel emptying.

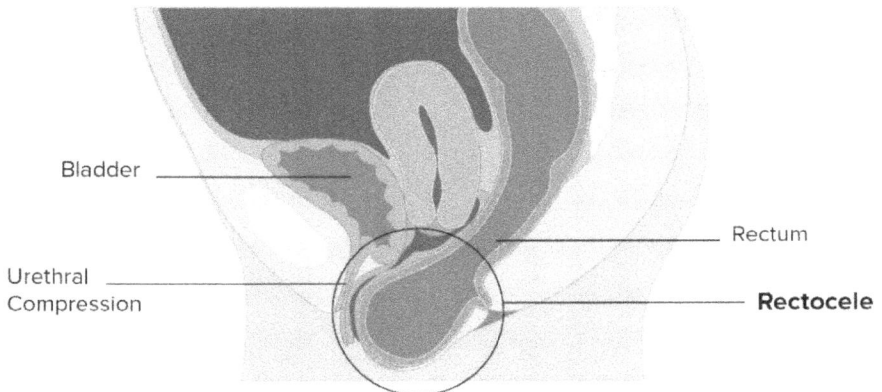

Rectocele. Image courtesy of Association for Pelvic Organ Prolapse Support.

Uterine

Uterine prolapse occurs when the uterus shifts downward through the vaginal canal. The uterus may rest inside but at the lower edge of the vagina; it can be completely within the vaginal walls or partially inside and outside of the vagina far enough for the cervix to be viewed outside of the vaginal opening. The most severe degree of uterine prolapse occurs when the uterus has pushed completely through the vaginal opening to the outside of the body. This condition is known as procidentia.

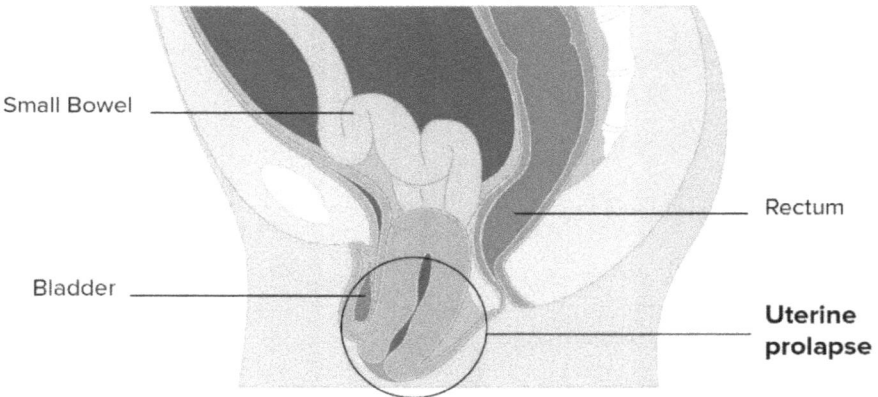

Uterine prolapse. Image courtesy of Association for Pelvic Organ Prolapse Support.

Vaginal Vault

The upper, inner portion of the vagina is known as the vaginal vault; it is also referred to as the apex. If the vaginal vault is not properly secured during hysterectomy, the vaginal walls may cave in on themselves and the vagina may invert, similar to turning a sock inside out. Vaginal tissue bulge and pressure are the most common symptoms of vaginal vault prolapse. Vaginal vault prolapse prevalence due to a hysterectomy varies considerably from study to study; the average prevalence rate is between 9% and 43%. However, repair techniques have evolved considerably. Although accurate data is difficult to confirm globally, this risk factor likely falls somewhere in the middle of the two figures.

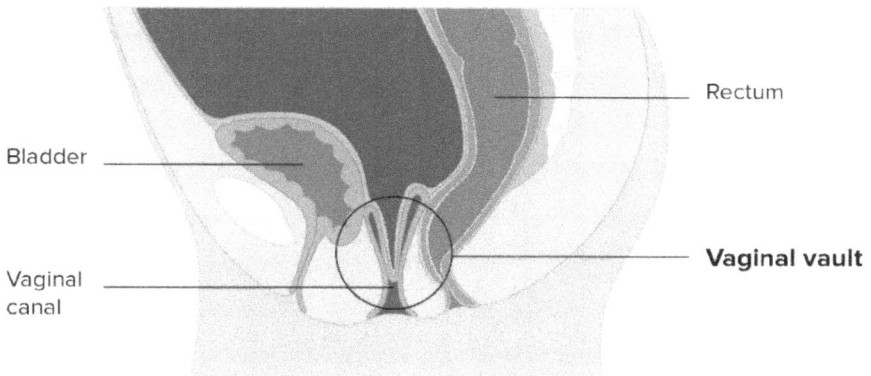

Vaginal Vault Prolapse. Image courtesy of Association for Pelvic Organ Prolapse Support.

Enterocele

An enterocele is a prolapse of the small bowel (intestines). An enterocele most characteristically occurs after a hysterectomy but can ensue as a result of a weakness in the membrane sack that contains intestines above the abdominal cavity. The intestines can push through any area of weakness in the sack, most typically in the apex (top of the vagina) where the uterus was formerly positioned. Intestines may push down between the rectum and the back wall of the vagina. They may also push down along the front vaginal wall. An enterocele rarely occurs alone; it often occurs simultaneously with a rectocele or vaginal vault prolapse.

As POP progresses and the organs and tissues shift and push against each other, the severity or complexity may be compounded. Early POP diagnosis is advantageous to contain the degree of severity and enable less aggressive treatment. Paying close attention to your body and knowing what is normal for you is key to early diagnosis and treatment.

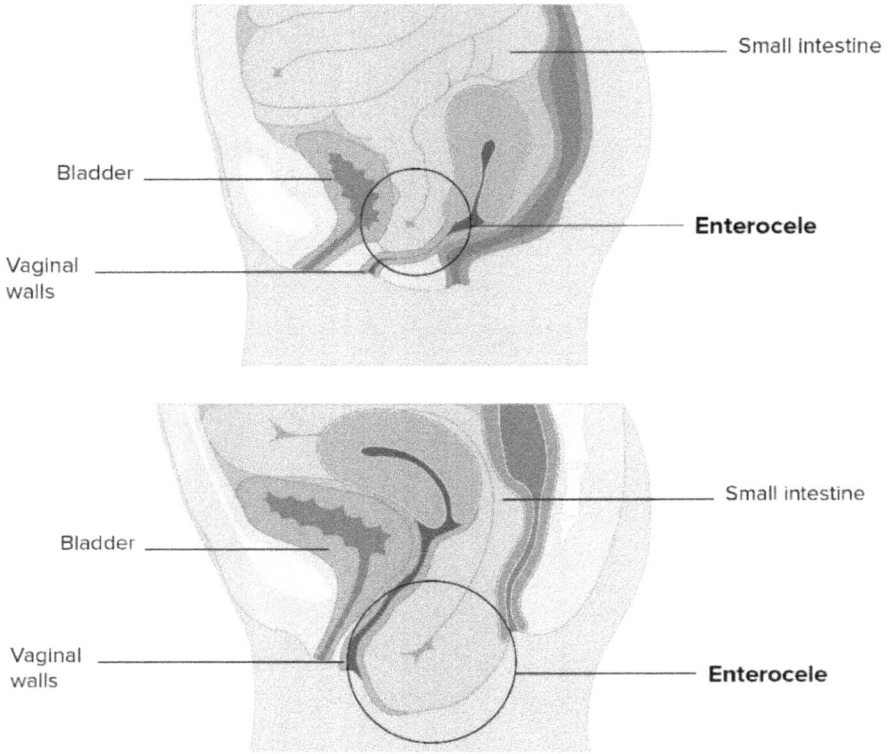

Image 1 enterocele in front of uterus, image 2 enterocele between vagina and rectum. Images courtesy of Association for Pelvic Organ Prolapse Support.

3

CAUSES OF PELVIC ORGAN PROLAPSE

APOPS Patient Perspective: *"APOPS is a sisterhood; we are no longer alone."*

~SK, Georgia/USA

I f there was a single cause of POP, it would be considerably easier to diagnose and treat. Unfortunately, there are numerous potential causes that may stand alone or piggyback each other. While POP causes have aspects of similarity among women, our somewhat distinct patterns of behavior and co-existing health concerns compound risk and severity in multiple ways. By its very multifaceted and at times ambiguous nature, POP often lingers unrecognized or misdiagnosed while continuing to degrade over time. Multiple factors or an isolated incident such as a difficult vaginal delivery may initiate POP.

While childbirth is considered the leading cause of POP, pregnancy in and of itself sets the stage. A considerable amount of strain is put on the support structures of the vagina and the pelvic floor throughout the gestation period.

"In my opinion this is one of the most important chapters in this excellent textbook. The causes of POP need to be widely disseminated to increase global awareness. Many of the causes highlighted include modifiable risk factors that women could address with lifestyle changes including improved diet and bowel function, weight loss, avoidance of heavy lifting in both the workplace and home as well

as an increasing acceptance of the benefits of HRT. Awareness of the importance of pelvic floor muscles in adulthood can form part of holistic body exercise programs and would make a significant impact in prevention of POP as one ages - prevention is better than cure."

Barry O'Reilly, MD

There are other factors that may contribute to POP occurrence or severity. While most women will have one primary causal factor, additional less prominent risk factors compound degree of symptom severity. The most commonly recognized POP causes include the following.

- Childbirth

- Estrogen depletion

- Genetic predisposition

- Tissue integrity

- Chronic constipation

- Chronic coughing

- Heavy lifting

- Obesity

- Hysterectomy

- Co-existing health conditions

- Diastasis rectus abdominus

- Adhesions and tissue damage

- High impact fitness activities

Childbirth

While having a baby is generally considered a joy-filled, momentous event, childbirth is the leading cause of POP. Childbirth can potentially damage pelvic floor muscles, nerves, and surrounding support tissues. Hormone levels fluctuate radically throughout pregnancy, delivery, and postpartum; this alters tissue integrity. Pressure and stretch applied to soft tissues during labor and childbirth amplify the potential for damage to occur.

Pelvic floor and surrounding soft tissues injured during delivery seldom recapture original tissue integrity or elasticity. When a woman has 2 or more deliveries within a short time frame and tissues haven't healed completely or properly from a prior delivery, the risk of prolapse is magnified. However, a period of rest between deliveries will not necessarily reduce the risk of POP.

Cesarean section (C-section) deliveries also come with the risk of POP occurring. Research indicates that elective C-section (no labor) results in less POP; however, an emergency C-section carries the risk of POP related to labor trauma that has already transpired. Surgical procedures that involve cutting into core structural tissues of the body may impact the underlying integrity of those tissues further down the road.

The two most common delivery factors that impact the likelihood of damage are prolonged labor and/or a large birth weight baby. When a woman gives birth, damage may occur to the levator ani muscle group (PC or pelvic floor muscle). The levator muscle group stretches from the pubic bone to the tailbone like a trampoline, supporting the organs above. This muscle bundle supports the uterus, bladder, and rectum. Sustained pressure from the baby's head on delicate tissues and nerve fibers in the vaginal canal during a lengthy 2nd stage of labor may cause long-term damage. Vacuum or suction delivery may also injure soft tissue structures including the PC. Damage may be obvious a short time after delivery; other times the impact might not be recognized for years, sometimes decades. Damage to the tissues and nerves in this area impacts the ability of the PC to contract. This makes it difficult to sustain support for the organs and the structural tissues that suspend them in position. Additionally, nerve or tissue damage may contribute to urinary or fecal incontinence.

An Oxford epidemiology study indicated that women experiencing vaginal childbirth twice were 8.4 times more likely to develop prolapse over women who had never experienced vaginal delivery. However, women who have never been pregnant may also develop POP since it has multiple causes.

Estrogen Depletion

Menopause is the 2nd leading cause of POP and is the most common reason for estrogen deficiency. Muscle tissue strength and integrity often drop when heading into menopause. However, it is important to note that there are multiple reasons for estrogen reduction, and it can occur in women during younger years as well. Additional causes of estrogen reduction may be chemotherapy, endocrine disorders, or congenital conditions.

When muscle tissue throughout the body weakens, regardless the cause, the structural integrity of both the pelvic floor and body core is impacted. As muscles, ligaments, and tendons lose density or strength, they can no longer sustain organs in position within the abdominal cavity. Good structural support for pelvic organs is critical in women to reduce the risk for and severity of POP.

Women may find benefits in hormone replacement therapy. HRT is often used to address diverse symptoms of perimenopause or menopause, whether utilizing traditional or bio-identically sourced hormones. Women who develop cancer are likely to experience menopausal-like estrogen depletion due to chemotherapy treatments. They are generally discouraged from using estrogen therapy. Hormone levels should be evaluated throughout cancer treatment regimens to assist diagnosis and management of estrogen loss ramifications, including POP.

Genetic Predisposition

As with other medical conditions, a genetic link may increase the risk of developing POP. Research indicates that chromosomes 10q and 17q may predispose women to POP. Recognition of symptoms is pivotal to early diagnosis and less aggressive treatment. Discussing symptoms with your mother, grandmothers, sisters, aunts, and cousins may provide insights into whether you have a POP predisposition.

It is quite possible that someone you are related to has had a POP procedure, but as is common with prolapse issues, it simply wasn't talked about. If someone in your family has had surgery related to this condition or incontinence, it may be beneficial to inquire what kind of treatments were provided.

Weak Tissue Integrity

Collagen is a protein that contributes to tissue elasticity and strength. Without sufficient levels of this protein, the pelvic floor structural components may weaken. Genetic factors that may come into play are hereditary diseases that impact tissue integrity.

Ehlers-Danlos syndrome (EDS) is a group of 13 connective tissue disorders that can be inherited and vary in their genetic composition. How they affect the body differs from person to person. Each EDS type manifests with unique genetic codes, with assorted insufficient amounts of structurally normal collagen. The primary complications seen in EDS involve the skin, muscles, skeleton, and blood vessels. The EDS/POP intersect is notable.

The most common types of EDS are characterized by joint hypermobility (joints that stretch further than normal), skin hyperextensibility (skin that stretches further than normal), and tissue fragility (easily bruises or tears). Structural tissues in women with EDS are less able to support organs effectively. EDS increases the risk of POP occurring and impacts treatment success. EDS co-existing with POP may reduce the benefit of nonsurgical treatments, increase the risk of surgical complications, or decrease potential for long-term surgical success.

Women who are "double-jointed" or have indicators of fragile tissue integrity should be mindful of POP symptoms whether or not they have given birth. This group of women includes adolescents who experience POP without having experienced pregnancy. Hard foot strike fitness activities such as gymnastics, running, or jogging may increase POP risk in EDS teenagers.

Marfan syndrome is another genetic disease evidenced by collagen deficiency. Women with EDS or Marfan should seek counsel with a genetic specialist or rheumatologist and a urogynecologist prior to surgery to discuss potential complications regarding lack of tissue integrity, which increases risk of surgical failure.

Chronic Constipation

Constipation is both a cause and a symptom of POP. Chronic constipation can have a significant impact on general health as well as pelvic organ and soft tissue placement within the pelvic cavity. When repetitively bearing down to have a bowel movement, the recurring pressure creating stress forces on all soft tissues and organs within the pelvic cavity and the rectum may cause or worsen POP.

Irritable bowel syndrome (IBS) is a relatively common condition that is often connected to stress that affects the large intestine. IBS causes symptoms such as cramping, abdominal pain, bloating, gas, diarrhea, constipation, or simultaneous diarrhea and constipation. IBS-related constipation may also contribute to POP.

A poor diet may also impact regularity. In today's fast-paced society, proper nutrition is often bypassed. We are frequently sleep deprived, don't take the time to exercise, and have little free time to relax after we address family and household concerns while typically punching out a forty+ hour work week.

Chronic Coughing

Smoking or living in a smoking household can lead to chronic coughing and multiple other health issues. Coughing can also be the result of allergies, emphysema, bronchitis, gastroesophageal reflux disease (GERD), poor air quality or inadequate ventilation, or insufficient air quality in the work environment. Chronic coughing triggers intra-abdominal pressure (IAP), a steady state of pressure within the abdominal cavity on soft support tissues and pelvic organs. The strain from chronic coughing can weaken support structures in the pelvic area. The repetitive jerking and downward displacement of organs can worsen POP.

Heavy Lifting

Everyone needs to lift heavy objects occasionally, but for some people, heavy lifting is continual or repetitive. Many occupations require heavy manual lifting; nursing, factory jobs, daycare, retirement home and rehabilitation facility staff, and farm workers are prime examples. Nearly all women who have children subject themselves to heavy lifting over and over. When our children hurt themselves and need comforting, we lift them. When we are rushed and the kids are taking too long to walk to where we want them to go, we lift them. When they are in trouble and we want to remove them from the scene of their activity, we lift them. When we put them into their car seats, shopping carts, bathtubs, or highchairs, we lift them. For women who have more than one small child, the motion is repetitious all day every day. Every time a woman lifts something heavy, intra-abdominal pressure is exerted within the pelvic cavity. Women are seldom aware that they should contract the pelvic floor or abdominal muscles prior to heavy lifting, so the pressure directly impacts core contents.

This is also true for women who weight train for health, muscle strength, or professional reasons. Women who are competitive weightlifting athletes are particularly prone to POP if not properly trained to protect the pelvic floor and core.

Obesity

Obesity has hit epidemic proportions in the US and can impact the degree of POP severity or treatment success. Excess weight may compound POP because of the constant pressure of abdominal fat on organs and structural tissues. Maintaining a healthy weight may help reduce the progression of POP.

Hysterectomy

According to the National Women's Health Network, approximately 600,000 hysterectomies are performed annually in the US.

Some women feel a strong emotional attachment to the uterus; others have so much pain and dysfunction with their reproductive anatomy that they are thrilled to explore surgical removal. Women suffering from POP symptoms who are seeking a direction to recapture QOL may choose a hysterectomy as a path to health ballast. Other times, hysterectomy is a surgical procedure that is utilized to address non-POP related health issues.

A health detail that is significant but insufficiently acknowledged is the uterus provides partial support to the top of the vagina. Studies indicate that the prevalence of vaginal vault prolapse following a hysterectomy will range between 0.2% to 43%. A hysterectomy may result in vaginal vault prolapse if the apex (top) of the vagina is not properly surgically secured simultaneously with the removal of the uterus. A hysterectomy will also increase the possibility of enterocele occurring. As is true of all surgeries, the hysterectomy technique utilized plays a role as does the skill of the surgeon providing the procedure.

Additionally, the uterus is a hub to the wagon wheel of organs around it. Organs in the pelvic cavity are positioned in proximity; if you remove the center hub, the surrounding organs may shift around the empty pocket to some degree. The potential for POP occurring post-hysterectomy is a concern of significance worth discussing with your surgeon.

Co-Existing Health Conditions

Neuromuscular diseases such as multiple sclerosis (MS) may increase the risk of POP. MS contributes to muscle weakness. When nerves can't fire properly, muscles tissues won't fully engage.

Bladder exstrophy is a congenital birth defect in which the bladder is open and exposed on the outside of the abdomen. The space inside the pelvic cavity predisposes women with exstrophy to POP.

Diabetes may be a concern since diabetics often suffer from neuropathy, which impacts how well nerves fire to initiate muscle contraction. Some degree of neuropathy contributing to pelvic floor disorders occurs in 11% to 67% of people with diabetes. When diseases cause paralysis or restriction of muscles or nerves, muscle tissue integrity deteriorates. The pelvic floor is deeply innervated muscle tissue; loss of nerve fire may reduce pivotal support to the pelvic organs.

Diastasis Rectus Abdominus

Another potential POP risk factor is diastasis rectus abdominus (DRA). This is a widening of the two bellies of the long abdominal muscle during pregnancy. While few studies validate that DRA increases the risk of urinary or fecal incontinence, myofascial pelvic pain, or pelvic organ prolapse, subjective feedback from women experiencing pelvic organ prolapse indicates that this is an area in need of research exploration.

Adhesions And Tissue Damage

Pelvic adhesions or scar tissue may occur in the soft tissues surrounding the bladder, bowel, or uterus. These tissue restrictions can result from infections, endometriosis, or prior surgery such as Cesarean deliveries. These tissue restrictions may continue to increase over time. They may limit structural tissue movement, compound POP symptoms, or complicate treatment.

Failure to repair structural support post-childbirth or during other abdominal or gynecologic surgeries can lead to tissue restriction that may later complicate POP treatment. Inadequate support of organs magnifies POP severity. Tissues torn during childbirth might not be recognized or repaired because the damage is internal. Injury may also occur to the nerves during the long 2nd stage of labor, which may affect the firing and function of muscle fibers and increase the risk of POP.

High-Impact Fitness Activities

Fitness activities are key to maintaining health balance, and millions of women participate in them. It is critical that POP awareness is increased in this sector of women. When participating in hard foot strike fitness activities, internal tissue support is critical to protect the pelvic floor and avoid trading one health concern for another.

There is notable potential for women who participate in hard foot strike fitness activities such as running, jogging, or gymnastics to experience POP. Studies indicate an estimated 18%-80% of young female athletes experience urinary leakage while exercising. Studies including both women who have given birth and those who had not reported an incontinence range from 45%-49%. Female marathon runners' primary complaint is not joint pain; it is incontinence, which is a common POP symptom. In 2021, 57% of runners in the US were women. The popularity of running continues to flourish for both fitness and stress relief.

In an ideal world, women would be advised that hard foot strike fitness activities impact pelvic floor support and increase the risk of leakage and prolapse. Less aggressive and equally beneficial fitness activities such as swimming or speed-walking provide safe muscle strengthening and aerobic benefits. However, due to endorphin and cardiovascular benefits, women are often committed to running or jogging.

Utilizing internal support such as a pessary is a pivotal proactive step all women who engage in more aggressive fitness activities should consider. While internal support is not a guarantee of POP prevention, it may reduce the risk of occurrence or severity. Inserting a pessary prior to high-impact athletic activities may reduce the impact of hard foot strike. Pessaries also reduce incontinence concerns when participating in athletic activities. It bears repeating, the most common complaint of female runners is not joint pain; it is urinary leakage.

Support garments may also provide a beneficial core and pelvic floor structural foundation for women engaging in more aggressive fitness activities. Research regarding support garments specifically developed to protect the pelvic floor is trending upward; more answers will soon become clear regarding their value.

4

SYMPTOMS OF PELVIC ORGAN PROLAPSE

APOPS Patient Perspective: *"The women in APOPS patient support space taught me more about my POP journey than the three specialists I saw combined. The information women share with each other in there is priceless, and I am so grateful to have found this priceless resource."*

~CC, Canada

Many women with POP have no idea there is a specific cause of the symptoms they experience. Some are too embarrassed to describe the symptoms to their physicians. Others are not in tune with their bodies and don't recognize that what they are experiencing is abnormal until the discomfort becomes too pronounced to ignore. Symptoms are often assumed to be an aspect of aging and are dismissed by clinicians as "normal" given a woman's age. At times, women are so busy they don't have or can't take the time to address their health issues at all.

For many women, POP symptoms come and go based on lifestyle, behaviors, activities, and co-existing health conditions. POP screening is not a standardized aspect of routine pelvic exams, and symptoms typically progress, especially if the condition has neither been screened for nor diagnosed.

*"Pelvic organ prolapse is an incredibly common and often embar-
rassing problem with pregnancy, labor, vaginal delivery, bowel "labor", and chronic increases in abdominal pressure as key risk factors.
In addition to altered genital anatomy giving rise to a variety of
symptoms as discussed in the chapter that follows, prolapse can also
lead to body dysmorphic disorder and a host of psychological and
emotional consequences. However, those suffering from pelvic organ
prolapse can rest assured that they are not alone, and that effective
guidance, support, treatments, and cure are possible."*

Andrew Siegel, MD

When lying down in supine position with feet in the stirrups (standard pelvic exam position), POP may not be clearly visible upon examination by clinicians who are not subspecialty trained in POP, or if POP is in a stage with a lower degree of severity. Additionally, the degree of POP severity may appear reduced lying down because organs tend to slide back into their normal position in the supine position.

Most diagnostic primary care physicians, gynecologists, and urologists refer patients experiencing POP to a subspecialist for further evaluation. A urogynecologist frequently uses a screening technique called POP-Q. This is an assessment in the distance of nine points in the vagina in relation to the position of the hymen, a thin, fleshy tissue located at the opening of the vagina. Primary care physicians and gynecologists are not trained in the POP-Q technique and more typically ask patients to perform a Valsalva maneuver (bearing down vaginally to visualize the degree of POP severity).

Because combinations of the five types of POP differs from woman to woman, symptoms may vary considerably from woman to woman. The degree of prolapse severity also fluctuates throughout the day because gravity drags organs downward when we are standing or engaging in upright activities. Women with a very mild degree of prolapse may not recognize symptoms at all or they may be very pronounced. POP symptoms may also replicate indicators of other conditions. The most common symptoms of POP are:

- Tissues bulging from the vagina

- Urinary incontinence

- Urine retention

- Chronic constipation

- Vaginal and/or rectal pressure

- Vaginal and/or rectal pain

- Back or pelvic pain

- Fecal incontinence

- Inability to retain a tampon

- Painful intercourse

- Reduced intimate sensation

The symptoms of POP can masquerade as or intersect with other disorders such as irritable bowel or generalized constipation from poor diet. Upon diagnosis of POP, a referral to a woman's health physical therapist or a urogynecologist is typically the next step to further evaluate and explore treatment options. The POP Risk Factor Questionnaire (POP-RFQ) is a self-screening tool available in the Appendix section of this book or in multiple languages via download from the Association for Pelvic Organ Prolapse (APOPS) website. The POP-RFQ clarifies whether symptoms being experienced indicate pelvic organ prolapse. This checklist may also help initiate a dialogue about POP with your clinician.

Tisssues Bulging Out Of The Vagina

The vaginal pressure that occurs with POP can be difficult to imagine without experiencing it. You may notice a bulge of tissue sitting just inside or minimally pushing outside of the vaginal canal. Some women describe this sensation as their insides falling out. Some say it feels like sitting on a ball. Others simply describe it as vaginal pressure.

The bulge of tissue exiting the vagina may indicate different types of POP manifestation. It could be the cervix, the opening to the uterus. It could be the uterus pushing out of the vaginal canal. It could be the vaginal wall with the bladder directly behind it. It could be the vaginal wall with the rectum directly behind it. It could be the vaginal wall with intestines directly behind it. If you have had a hysterectomy, it could be the apex (top) of the vaginal walls caving in on themselves and collapsing completely through the vaginal canal to the outside of the body. This sitting-on-a-ball sensation may come and go because prolapsed organs can shift back into the pelvic cavity. Women who are on their feet all day because of their jobs or childcare may not recognize POP for some time because they are distracted by everyday activities and are rarely aware the condition exists before being diagnosed. Since pelvic organs can retract into their normal position when a woman lies down in bed at night, she may no longer feel any pain or discomfort.

Some women push the bulging tissues back up into the vaginal canal to relieve the pressure. While it is safe to do so (wash your hands first!), this is a temporary fix that relieves the sensation or may enable urination or defecation.

Urinary Incontinence

Urinary incontinence (UI) is often considered a condition, but it is also one of the most common symptoms of POP. While incontinence issues are not always POP related, there is a notable POP connection. Millions of women suffer from UI, and most do not seek medical evaluation. Women with UI often believe it is a normal part of aging; they don't recognize it is a symptom of a health condition that must be diagnosed and addressed. Studies indicate that 25% of young women, 44% to 57% of middle-aged and post-menopausal women, and 75% of elderly women in nursing homes experience some level of urinary incontinence.

Urinary incontinence manifests in various forms. The primary categories are stress urinary incontinence (SUI), urge urinary incontinence (UUI), overactive bladder (OAB), and mixed urinary incontinence (MUI).

Stress urinary incontinence (SUI) occurs when the bladder leaks urine during physical activities that increase intra-abdominal pressure. The causes can be as simple as sneezing, coughing, or laughing. They may be related to lifestyle and activities such as fitness or intimacy.

When SUI occurs during hard foot strike or heavy lifting athletic or fitness activities, it is called athletic urinary incontinence (AUI). Women are very active in today's society. Fitness benefits our health, stress reduction, social engagement, and self-esteem. Running and jogging are hugely popular fitness activities, as are fitness center memberships that provide diverse fitness options. However, hard foot strike and heavy lifting fitness activities, while improving health in various ways, can be detrimental to female pelvic floor health. Incontinence occurring during these activities is a clear indicator of the impact of hard foot strike activities or intra-abdominal pressure occurring when lifting heavy weight.

I'm a fitness geek; I get it. But it is critical to modify the types of fitness activities we engage in to better protect and preserve our pelvic floor health.

Coital incontinence (CUI) is a form of SUI urine leakage that may occur during penetration of intercourse, masturbation, or orgasm. Reportedly, it occurs in 10%-27% of sexually active women with urinary incontinence concerns.

Urge urinary incontinence is the result of bladder spasms that create a strong, sudden need to urinate that is difficult to delay and results in urine leakage. Urge urinary incontinence can result from a urinary tract infection (UTI), bladder inflammation or stones, nerve injury, bladder cancer, or hormone fluctuation around the time of menopause. It can also occur when pressure is exerted on pelvic organs related to the bearing down during bowel movements, as often occurs in those experiencing frequent constipation, common with a rectocele.

OAB is a repetitive urge to urinate immediately without leakage. It occurs when muscles that control bladder function act up involuntarily, causing a frequent or sudden urge to urinate that may be difficult to manage. OAB causes may be related to diseases such as stroke, multiple sclerosis (MS) or diabetes. OAB can also be related to nerve damage, medications, alcohol or caffeine use, infection, or being overweight.

Mixed urinary incontinence is any combination of types of urinary leakage.

Urinary incontinence is more typical in the early stages of prolapse. As POP advances to a more pronounced stage, voiding difficulties and incomplete emptying become more frequent or more pronounced. Remember, not all incontinence is due to prolapse, so it is critical to consult with a physician for an accurate diagnosis. Urinary incontinence occurs frequently in women after childbirth because of trauma to the pelvic floor structural support tissues and nerves or hormone fluctuations. If urinary incontinence does not resolve after childbirth (especially if you experienced a difficult labor), it is important to request an evaluation.

Urine Retention

Often women who have incontinence in early stages of prolapse have difficulty voiding effectively later in a more advanced stage. When POP has progressed to grade 3 or 4, urine retention, a weak urine stream, or difficulty emptying the bladder completely may occur. With advanced cystocele, the urethra may kink (the tube through which urine passes from the bladder to the outside of the body). This makes it difficult for the bladder to empty. If urine cannot flow from the body effectively or fully, there is an increased risk of urinary tract infections (UTI).

One study indicates obstruction of the urethra occurred in 58% of women with grades 3 & 4 prolapse. In comparison, only 4% of women with grade 1 or 2 prolapse experienced obstruction of the urethra. As the degree of prolapse progresses, it is more likely that a woman will have difficulty initiating the urine stream. It may be necessary to manually reduce the prolapse with finger or hand pressure on abdomen, perineum, or inside of the vagina to void urine.

Chronic Constipation

Although constipation has many causes, chronic constipation is a common indicator of POP in women. When the hernia bulge of a rectocele balloons out from the colon, it prevents stool from passing normally through the bowel. Constipation can occur on and off in early stages of POP. Typically it becomes a daily occurrence in moderate to advanced stages of rectocele. There may be a need to "splint" to enable defecation. This involves inserting two fingers into the vagina to push against the rear vaginal wall to encourage a bowel movement – additionally worth repeating - always wash hands before inserting fingers into the vagina. IBS may also cause constipation, so it is important to have a practitioner evaluate bowel concerns.

Stool incontinence may occur simultaneously with chronic constipation in women with POP. Since rectocele constipation is caused by this hernia-like bulge in the rectum, a high-fiber diet may not eliminate the problem. Increasing water intake, supplementing with probiotics, and using produce rather than grain fiber sources sometimes helps. However, is typically difficult to relieve POP-related constipation. POP treatments are also necessary to reduce symptoms.

Vaginal And/Or Rectal Pressure

Vaginal or rectal pressure is difficult to explain to someone who has not experienced it. The "fullness" that accompanies pressure in these areas may lead to an incorrect diagnosis or less than clarifying diagnostic test. Women who are used to period bloating, the distended feeling that accompanies PMS, may misinterpret this sensation. POP pressure is typically most pronounced specifically in the rectum or vagina.

Nearly everyone is familiar with the urge sensation of rectal pressure that is felt when a bowel movement is coming on. For a woman with a rectocele, a bowel movement may only minimally or temporarily relieve the urge or pressure sensation.

Vaginal And/Or Rectal Pain

Since pain is unique from person to person, it is important to note that one woman may perceive rectal or vaginal fullness as pressure, another may perceive it as pain. The level of discomfort that grows with each day of not being able to properly empty your bowels can be very stressful. If a woman believes she has IBS or typical constipation and tries several remedies to no avail, it would be worthwhile exploring whether other POP symptoms are occurring. If so, a POP exploration to establish POP diagnosis and treatment is appropriate.

Back And/Or Pelvic Pain

Because there can be multiple combinations of organs and tissues involved with POP, the type and degree of pain experienced differs from woman to woman. At times, pain can radiate to the lower back. Pressure pain may occur in the rectum or vagina. Generalized pelvic distention may cause pain. Discomfort may feel similar to a urinary tract infection. Pain may occur with intercourse, and a general heaviness may occur throughout the pelvic region. POP pain and discomfort often ease when lying down. Not all pelvic pain is related to POP. It is important to keep track of all symptoms to clarify if the pain is genuinely POP associated.

Fecal Incontinence

It is estimated that up to 40% of women will sustain some damage to the sphincter muscle or its nerve supply during childbirth. After obstetrical anal injury and repair, 50% of women continue to experience some degree of bowel incontinence, more commonly referred to as fecal incontinence (FI). FI may not show up until decades after childbirth. When this occurs, women seldom recognize the connection between FI and childbirth experiences long past.

Inability To Retain A Tampon

One indicator of POP that may occur before any other symptom is recognized is the inability to keep a tampon in place. Normally when a tampon is inserted into the vagina, soft tissues and muscular structures naturally hold it in position.

When POP occurs, the altered position of organs and tissues literally push the tampon downward into or out of the vagina. If experiencing tampon expulsion, review the APOPS POP-RFQ questionnaire in the Appendix section of this book and request POP screening from your primary care physician or gynecologist.

Coital Incontinence

Incontinence is enough to completely put the skids on romance; it can take the spontaneity out of intimacy. Most people aren't comfortable talking about incontinence. It's even more difficult to approach the topic of incontinence related to intimacy, especially fecal incontinence. Any woman who must worry if she will remain "clean" during sexual activity will generally avoid being spontaneous.

Since there is a possibility of stool or urine leakage with POP, women may refrain from sexual relations out of fear that these issues may occur. It is rare that a woman will explain this to her partner ahead of the curve. Women often find it uncomfortable to talk about stool or urine leakage with even the closest partner. As a result, one partner may believe the other partner is not interested in sex when the reality is that the issue is a medical condition that has not been acknowledged, diagnosed, or treated.

Painful Intercourse

POP displacement of organs may cause sexual pain or discomfort. Rather than reveal that intercourse is painful, a woman may choose to indicate she is not interested in sex. Others share that intercourse is painful, but their partners do not always believe them, especially if this occurs regularly.

Sometimes struggles with intimacy are what bring POP to the front page. When a woman who has enjoyed sex her entire adult life suddenly finds intimacy painful, confusion and frustration can occur. A woman may assume the changes are due to typical aging changes rather than something more significant. While vaginal atrophy (thinning, drying and/or irritation of the vaginal walls related to estrogen loss) is very real, not all pain with intimacy is related to atrophy. A clinician may check hormone levels to determine whether estrogen replacement may address intimate pain related to atrophy. If pain continues after atrophy has been addressed, the pressure of POP organ displacement or related abdominal bloat may be the source of discomfort.

Reduced Intimate Sensation

Nerve damage or stretching of soft tissues resulting from childbirth may reduce or prevent sensation from reaching areas that were previously sexually sensitive. Lack of intimate sensation compounds self-esteem struggles that women experience when navigating tissues bulging out of the vagina. If there is little or no sensation during foreplay or intercourse, a woman may lose interest in intimacy. This loss of intimacy can clearly have a detrimental impact on a relationship.

Most women struggle to discuss intimate sensations with their physicians or their sexual partners. Intimacy conversations are often awkward to initiate whether they have medical, physical, or emotional roots. However, these concerns can and should be examined and openly discussed.

Fecal incontinence, athletic incontinence, coital incontinence, painful intercourse, reduced intimate sensation, and vaginal tissue bulge can radically impact an intimate relationship between the sexually active woman and her partner. Open communication in a relationship is ideal but not common when it comes to concerns of this delicate nature.

Telling an intimate partner about any of the above concerns is difficult enough. However, lack of info share can lead them to assume there is no interest in intimacy at all. Experiencing a partner's assumption, these are excuses to get out of being intimate can be hurtful and frustrating, destructive to a relationship. Initiating a conversation, as difficult as it may be, may ease tensions.

TESTS AND TREATMENTS: ANALYZING OPTIONS

5

MEDICAL EVALUATION: WHAT TO EXPECT

APOPS Patient Perspective: *"Because of APOPS, I found the strength to say this isn't normal and I can do something about it - to myself and to my doctors."*

~MO, Georgia/USA

Prior to being clinically diagnosed with the type(s) and grade of POP severity, pelvic organ prolapse is typically initially diagnosed by a gynecologist or primary care practitioner. Nonsurgical treatments may be recommended by your primary physician, such as Kegel exercises or a pessary, or sometimes a combination of the two. The next step may be referral to a physical therapist specializing in women's health to enable the patient to better understand the pelvic floor and what types of self-care or treatments may reduce the degree of POP severity or symptoms. Alternatively, women may be referred to a urogynecologist for evaluation. Sometimes women's health PTs and urogynecologists work hand in hand to address patient needs in an integrated healthcare system.

Bring your list of symptoms and questions to the exam appointment and a notebook to take notes to review later. After discussing the reason for your visit and reviewing your symptoms, a urogynecologist will most likely perform both a vaginal and rectal exam to make an initial determination regarding the type(s) of prolapse you have and the degree of severity.

*"The diagnostic process of a woman with POP is not just to exe-
cute some examinations taken from a list. One should consider the
anatomical defects and the correlated symptoms, keep in mind the
possible pathophysiology together with the patient's real aims and ex-
pectations, and make all the evaluations needed. Sometimes taking
a history and a physical examination may be enough, sometimes in-
strumental examinations may be needed. The patient's needs should
rule this process, always."*

Enrico Finazzi-Agro, MD

A good practitioner will explain what they are doing before performing each part
of the exam. If you do not have a good comfort level with your physician during
this exam, it will surely not get any better once you get to the point of surgery. If at
any point you feel your practitioner is not explaining in advance what is going to
be done, speak up. If you experience pain during any part of the exam, speak up. If
you have a question, speak up. If your practitioner is gentle and concerned about
the sensitive nature of this exam, it is an indicator that you have a compassionate
subspecialist. Patients often hesitate to ask questions because they feel physicians
are busy and they don't want to slow them down, or the questions they have are
embarrassing to bring up. You are paying for this medical service, whether out
of your own pocket or paying for the insurance coverage. View it like any other
service, expect the best.

The initial vaginal inspection by a subspecialist will be similar to the traditional
pelvic exam that occurs with your gynecologist or primary care physician, lying on
your back with the feet in stirrups, hips and knees flexed, legs spread. By visually
inspecting and palpating each wall of the vagina with a single blade speculum
while you cough and bear down vaginally (Valsalva maneuver), in addition to
palpating the abdominal area, a subspecialist will determine which organ zones
are prolapsing.

The Pelvic Organ Prolapse Quantification System (POP-Q) is a technique to
assess the degree of prolapse, enabling a urogynecologist to determine the degree
of POP severity. When assessing POP prevalence using the POP-Q, the incidence
of pelvic organ prolapse is estimated to be up to 50%. Some studies indicate that
POP diagnosis by symptoms alone interprets a much lower prevalence. Considering women find POP symptoms embarrassing and may not admit to some of
them, the low prevalence referenced by symptoms alone is very likely far from
accurate.

The POP-Q defines the severity of prolapse between grades 1, 2, 3, or 4, grade 1 being the mildest prolapse, grade 4 being the most severe. A grade 1 prolapse may not cause any symptoms. Grade 2 can be extremely variable, from very mild symptoms to relatively acute symptoms. In grade 2 there is typically some degree of tissue bulge visible in the vaginal opening or organs/vaginal tissue minimally protruding out of the vagina. When standing, the tissue bulge is more pronounced. By grade 3, the physical symptoms are not only felt by the patient, but they are also typically quite pronounced and the prolapse is clearly visible. At the point of grade 4, symptoms and vaginal tissue bulge are substantial. If a woman has uterine prolapse, grade 4 means her uterus is completely outside of her body (procidentia). Despite apparent symptoms, POP may go undiagnosed for years, sometimes decades, because POP evaluation is not a standardized aspect of women's wellness checks, women are too embarrassed to share their symptoms with their primary care physicians or gynecologists, and these physicians are not sufficiently educated about POP to screen appropriately.

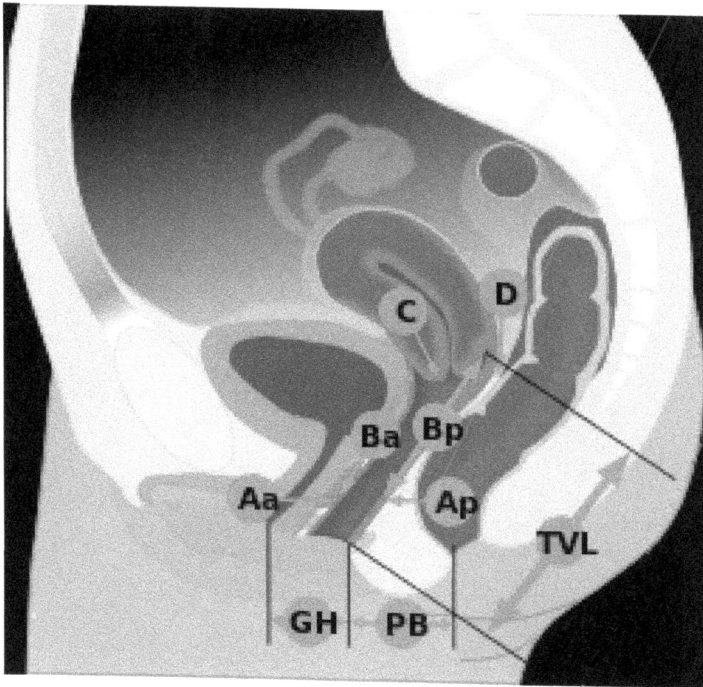

POP-Q exam. Image courtesy of Wikipedia.

During a rectal exam, the physician will insert a lubricated, gloved finger into the rectum and may possibly insert fingers from the other hand into the vagina. The physician will ask you to bear down as if having a bowel movement to assess how far down the vaginal canal the organs have shifted. It is a relatively quick check with minimal discomfort.

Besides visually inspecting the vagina both with and without a speculum, a urogynecologist may also check the strength of the pubococcygeus contraction (better known as a Kegel, a PC contraction, or a pelvic floor muscle contraction). During the vaginal exam, the practitioner will insert fingers manually and ask you to squeeze or tighten your pelvic floor muscles as if you're stopping a stream of urine to check the strength of your PC. A Kegel contraction is up and in, as opposed to a Valsalva maneuver pushing down and out. It is important during this test to pull up and in rather than bear down as though having a bowel movement.

After the POP-Q exam has been completed and you have a preliminary diagnosis regarding type/types of POP, additional diagnostic tests may be required to clarify issues that need to be addressed. Tests that may be performed to clarify POP or additional health concerns are:

- The Standing Screen

- Urodynamic Study

- 3D Pelvic Ultrasound

- Hormone Level Analysis

- Cystoscopy

- Defecography MRI

- 3D Endoanal Ultrasound

- Abdominal/Pelvic CT Scan

- Biomechanical Mapping

The Standing Screen

Prolapse severity is reduced when laying on your back in lithotomy position, so in addition to being examined in that position, you may be examined standing. No speculum is used during standing exams; hand palpation is the screening method. If your physician screens in the lithotomy position and indicates the degree of

POP severity is mild but your symptoms indicate otherwise, request the standing screen if it is not offered to you.

Urodynamic Study

Your physician may want bladder tests prior to surgery even if you are not experiencing leakage issues. In more advanced cases of POP, prolapse may mask urinary incontinence because the prolapsed organs or tissues may press against and create a kink in the urethra, the tube through which urine flows from the bladder to the outside of the body, preventing urine from leaking out. Once the POP issues are repaired and the urethra is no longer kinked, you may discover that you now have a urine leakage problem. Urinary incontinence is common in women. It makes sense to test for incontinence concerns prior to surgery so leakage you aren't aware of, which can occur in advanced degrees of POP severity, can be addressed at the same time as POP surgery.

Urodynamics is a group of tests to determine how well the bladder stores and empties urine. It provides information regarding how much the bladder can hold before there is an urge to urinate, how well the bladder muscle functions, whether there might be a sphincter or pelvic floor dysfunction hindering the outflow of urine, and whether urine remains in your bladder after it feels like you're finished urinating.

The amount and force of the urine stream are measured in the first portion of the test. A catheter is inserted for the second part of the test and the bladder is filled with sterile water. A measurement is taken for the volume at which the patient feels the need to urinate. The patient is then asked to bear down and cough to see if urine leaks out. This test also determines bladder flow and bladder pressure at the time of urinating. The results of this test help the surgeon determine the best type of surgical repair.

3D Pelvic Ultrasound

3D pelvic ultrasound provides imagery of the pelvic organs, soft tissues, pelvic floor muscles, and perineum to assess issues related to POP, fecal incontinence, or trauma resulting from childbirth or prior pelvic surgeries. Ultrasound imagery is captured via transabdominal, perineal, transrectal or translabial probes to clarify issues with clarity and absence of distortion. Various transducer heads (probes) produce sound waves when inserted into the vaginal or rectal cavity that bounce off body tissues and make echoes, sending them to a computer to create an image called a sonogram.

This 3D imagery includes a multitude of sectional planes within the pelvic cavity, including the midsagittal (right and left sides), coronal (front and rear), and axial (viewing from all angles around the center of the object being viewed). The probes can capture imaging of a pc contraction (contracting in and up) and Valsalva maneuver (bearing down), vaginal or rectal wall abnormalities, anal sphincter damage, fistula, or visualization of tapes and meshes used to repair prolapse and incontinence.

Hormone Level Analysis

Estrogen is a source of female tissue strength and integrity. Hormone testing is a blood test that clarifies levels circulating in the body. Female hormone levels can be checked to determine whether estrogen loss is contributing to pelvic floor weakness. Menopause is research validated as the 2nd leading cause of POP, but women navigating cancer treatment regardless the age are often hormone depleted as well as a result of chemotherapy or other cancer treatments. If a woman is already on hormone replacement therapy, this test may not be necessary. Women who have not used hormone therapies and are in menopause should consider requesting a check of hormone levels prior to surgery since loss of estrogen can impact the capacity for tissue to heal post-surgery. Physicians may recommend temporary hormone supplementation for women in perimenopause or menopause who are not already utilizing hormone therapy to enhance the healing of the vaginal and pelvic floor tissues.

Cystoscopy

Cystoscopy is a test that views inside the bladder and urethra. It may be necessary to evaluate bladder pain or blood in the urine prior to surgery. A small tube with a light and camera are lubricated with an anesthetic gel and inserted into the urethra; images are projected onto a screen for viewing.

Defecography MRI

Magnetic resonance imaging (MRI) defecography captures images of various stages of defecation to evaluate how well colon and rectal muscles are working to provide insight into the rectum's ability to defecate normally. Defecography shows the rectum and anal canal in action while having a bowel movement by the insertion of a barium paste into the rectum. You'll evacuate the paste in the same way as having a bowel movement on a special toilet behind a curtain while the radiologist monitors your internal tissue activity on a computer screen. Weak rectal walls will bulge out as a hernia clarifying rectocele location, and the grade of severity can be clarified.

3D Endoanal Ultrasound

Obstetric anal sphincter injuries (OASIS) are complications that can occur to the rectal sphincter during a vaginal delivery. Sphincter tears can be an unrecognized, unresolved aspect of childbirth damage. Even when identified post-birthing, they may not be properly repaired, resulting in long-term discomfort and rectal dysfunction. 3D endoanal ultrasound is an imaging tool that can clarify damage or identify repair failures. An endoanal US can also evaluate and grade rectal sphincter atrophy.

Abdominal/Pelvic CT Scan

Both MRIs and CT scans can view internal body structures such as bones, cartilage, muscles, tendons, and organs. A CT scan is faster and quieter; MRIs are more detailed in their imaging.

Biomechanical Mapping

A vaginal tactile imager (VTI) achieves high-resolution mapping of pressures of soft tissues within the vaginal canal and assesses the strength of the pelvic floor muscles. This device can assist diagnosis and evaluation of how the vaginal walls react to pressures pushing against them along the entire vaginal canal. VTI records pelvic floor muscle contraction patterns and assesses tissue elasticity and pelvic floor support, with a focus on pelvic organ prolapse, urinary incontinence, and tissue atrophy in women.

Upon completion of testing, your physician will determine the treatment which will provide the best options, whether surgical or non-surgical. These tests enable urogynecologists to precisely determine the types and severity of POP, increasing the potential for all prolapsed organs to be repaired in one surgical procedure.

6

NONSURGICAL TREATMENT OPTIONS

APOPS Patient Perspective: "*One of the greatest challenges women with POP face is how isolating it is. APOPS gave me the strength to recognize that educating myself about this highly stigmatized condition would enable me to grow strong and empowered to move forward with appropriate health care decisions. With this sisterhood, I no longer feel alone. I am so grateful for Sherrie Palm and APOPS efforts.*"

~BR, Oregon/USA

There are two treatment paths for POP, surgical or nonsurgical. No woman needs to have surgery for pelvic organ prolapse or any other health condition; it is always patient choice. After your primary care physician or gynecologist has diagnosed POP, a subspecialist can guide your treatment path. Each treatment option has its distinct benefits and the choice you make will be influenced by your type and grade of POP, whether or not you choose to have a child or additional children, the length of time you have been suffering with symptoms, the severity of your symptoms, complications your unique co-existing medical conditions may pose, your age, your desire to continue to have sexual relations, and medical insurance coverage considerations.

A variety of POP health practitioners can guide you through the nonsurgical treatment options. Treatments provided by therapists provide POP symptom nonsurgical management rather than surgical repair, and these therapies additionally have benefits for maintenance post-surgery. Make sure the therapists you choose are certified in women's pelvic health.

Becoming more aware of your body and the sensations POP causes will be of great value in monitoring your path to pelvic and pelvic floor health balance. Many women with grades 1 or 2 POP find combinations of the following treatments effective to control POP symptoms and may relieve degree of symptom bother in grade 3 POP. Additionally, these treatments can be rebooted for long-term maintenance post-surgery should the surgical route be your treatment choice.

- Pessary

- Impressa

- Kegel Exercises

- PC Strengthening Devices

- Pelvic Floor and Core Exercise Programs

- Hormone Replacement Therapy

- Nonsurgical Vaginal Rejuvenation

- Emsella Chair

- Support Garments

- Vaginal Electrical Stimulation

- Tibial Nerve Stimulation

- Biofeedback

- Urethral Bulking Agents

- Myofascial Release Therapy

Any combination of these approaches may be used, depending on the type or types of prolapse experienced. Your healthcare professionals will guide your exploration of a combination of therapies to improve pelvic floor health. These therapies may reduce POP symptoms and if utilized routinely and appropriately, may reduce potential for an additional increase in POP severity. It will generally take a few months for these types of therapies to produce benefit, and they must be continued to maintain the benefit.

Pessary

Prior to being diagnosed with pelvic organ prolapse, I had never heard of a pessary. Once again, I was amazed that despite researching various women's health issues that wandered across my line of vision and openly discussing health topics with my practitioners, I had not only never heard of pelvic organ prolapse, but I'd also never heard of a pessary. I wondered how pessary use got past my women's health radar; it's not like I live in a cave.

While I started gathering survey data in the early years of my exploration of the POP pathway to capture intel whether women I knew had heard of pelvic organ prolapse, I also routinely inquired whether they had ever heard of a pessary. I discovered that the two topics go hand in hand; those who knew about POP knew about pessaries; those unfamiliar with POP were in the dark.

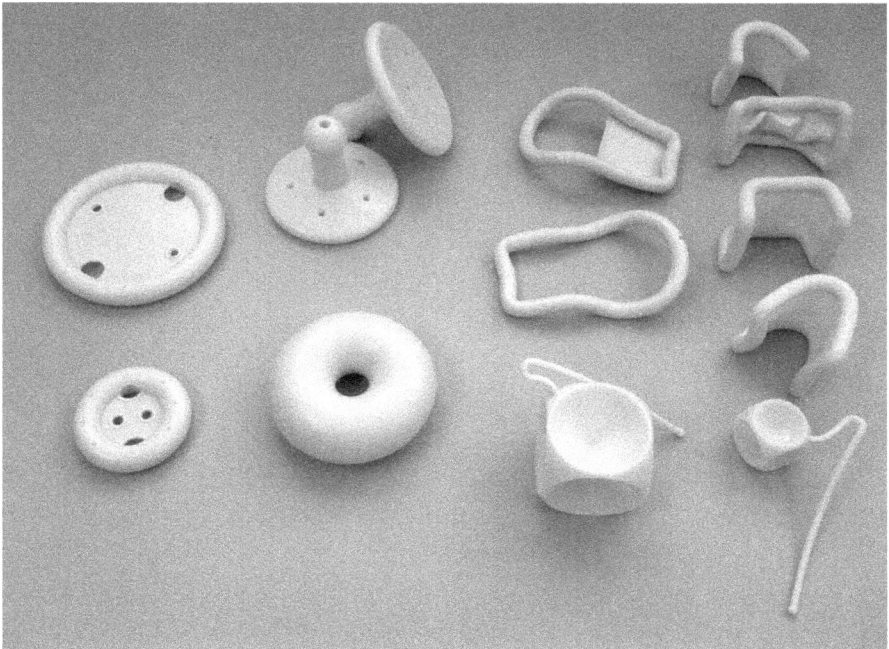

Pessary. Image courtesy of Wikipedia.

Pessaries are man-made devices with Latin and Greek origins dating back prior to Hippocrates era, documented in Egyptian papyruses. The mechanical devices from ancient times are very unlike the modern versions. Honey, wine, hot oil, fumes, and pomegranates (Hippocrates's pessary choice) were commonly used. In the middle-ages, a ball of linen or wool soaked in diverse potions was the treatment of choice. Eventually, pessary design progressed and began to resemble the pessaries of today.

The modern pessary is a silicone nonsurgical medical device (in some developing countries, latex pessaries are also still used) that is vaginally inserted to support prolapsed organs, and is often the first line of treatment offered to women. A pessary is somewhat similar in dimension/design to a contraceptive diaphragm and is available in a variety of shapes and sizes since each woman's internal structure is somewhat unique. The most commonly prescribed types of pessaries used are ring, ring with support, donut, Gellhorn, Gehring, and Cube, but there are over 20 styles of pessaries currently available and additional designs in development. Pessaries should be fitted by a clinician to ensure the best type and fit. The particular type of pessary used will depend on the type(s) of prolapse and grade of POP severity.

A pessary can decrease the symptoms of POP and may provide an option to temporarily delay or avoid surgery. In some instances, a pessary may prevent POP from progressing. Other potential benefits of a pessary are:

- Treatment for women who are not candidates for surgery.

- Surgical delay for financial reasons, lack of childcare assistance, work conflicts, or waiting for health insurance deductible to be reached.

- High risk of surgical complications related to advanced age or medical co-morbidities.

- Waiting to complete childbearing prior to surgical repair.

- Incontinence evaluation to see if urinary leakage should be addressed at the same time as prolapse repair.

- Controlling incontinence during fitness activities.

- Maintaining pregnancy in women with uterine prolapse.

- Determining whether surgery will bring relief of symptoms that do not match the physical findings.

If you intend to use a pessary, it is important to inform your physician about latex allergies. Silicone pessaries have the advantage of being anti-allergenic; they do not absorb secretions or odors, stay pliable and soft, and retain their integrity after repeated cleanings daily for years.

Pessaries can be divided into two categories, support and space-filling. Women come in all shapes and sizes, both internally and externally. Support pessaries are typically used for grades 2 or 3 POP while space-filling pessaries are more typically used for grades 3 or 4. Some pessaries have holes in their design to allow secretions to pass through since the pessary may be left in place for extended periods of time.

If a pessary is too small, it will not provide adequate support, or it may pop out of place. If it is too large, it will be uncomfortable and may cause tissue erosion. You may need to experiment with a few different sizes or types of pessaries at your physician's office before a correct type and size is fitted that feels comfortable and stays in place.

For the fitting itself, your physician will initially insert a pessary based on the type and size they think you may need. You will be asked to squat, sit, walk around, cough, and bear down to see if the pessary stays in position. Do not hesitate to let your physician know if the pessary feels uncomfortable, causes pain, or feels too loose, even if it is the second, third, or fourth pessary tried. It is important to get the correct pessary type and fit so you can continue to wear it comfortably. When a pessary fits properly, you should not feel it, much like a tampon.

Once you and your physician find the appropriate pessary for your needs, you will be asked to make a follow-up appointment within a few days to a month to enable your physician to recheck the pessary to assure it is working properly and not creating any irritations, allergic reactions, or pressure sores. If prior to your next appointment you experience tissue irritation, excessive vaginal discharge, pain, if the pessary pops out, if you can't empty your bladder, if bleeding occurs, or if the pessary you have been given no longer feels "right", contact your physician's office immediately to have the pessary checked. Your physician may need to insert a different size or type of pessary. Do not wait for your follow-up appointment if this occurs, do it right away or tissue irritation may occur or progress, and pessary use may need to be discontinued until the tissues are healed. The most common complaint with pessary use is discomfort, which indicates you may have been fitted with the wrong size or type.

Some pessaries can be inserted, removed, cleaned, and reinserted by the patient themselves. Others must be routinely maintained by your clinician. I highly recommend letting your physician instruct you how to insert and remove your own pessary when possible. Leaving a pessary in 24 hours a day increases risk of tissue erosion. To optimize vaginal tissue health, pessaries that patients can insert at the start of their day and remove prior to going to bed are the most beneficial option, allowing the tissues time to breathe pessary-free overnight.

Inserting and removing your own pessary will enable you to proactively control prolapse symptoms in the event you don't want or need to use your pessary all the time. Women who use a pessary while engaging in a fitness activity may only want to insert it during those more active time slots. After a short period of use, it will be easy to decide whether you will be able to tolerate using a pessary long term or if you will eventually want surgery for a more permanent fix.

Most clinicians who fit pessaries will instruct you how to insert and remove your pessary while you are being fitted. It takes a bit of practice to get comfortable using a pessary, similar to the learning curve necessary with contact lenses for vision correction. In the beginning, it seems to take forever for insertion, but in a very short time, the insertion and removal process is fast and relatively easy.

It is important to follow your physician's instructions regarding care of your pessary. Some may be worn for days to weeks (in some cases months) at a time, but from personal experience I highly recommend daily removal and reinsertion when possible.

Some women may not be comfortable with the idea of inserting their own pessary; others simply don't want to be bothered. If this is the case, let your physician know at your fitting, as this will impact the type of pessary they choose for you. If you won't be removing your own pessary, your clinician will need to remove it for cleaning minimally once every three months. At that time, your clinician can also check for any ulcerations or irritations.

There is a possibility that you may need to use a vaginal estrogen cream to prevent erosions of the vaginal tissues from the pressure of your pessary rubbing, especially if you are experiencing any perimenopausal or menopausal vaginal tissue atrophy.

If you notice a foul-smelling discharge, the vaginal acid balance needs to be restored. An acidic vaginal gel such as Trimo-San will reduce tissue sensitivity and odor. Women who are post-menopausal whose vaginal tissues are very thin and dry may need to use both an estrogen cream and the acidic vaginal gel.

There are a few reasons women won't be able to use a pessary:

- Frequent infections or irritations of the vaginal tissues.

- Pelvic inflammatory disease.

- Unwilling or unable to perform necessary maintenance, whether self-maintenance or practitioner maintenance.

- Unwilling or unable to get to the physician's office for routine checkups.

- Latex allergy or silicone sensitivity.

- Advanced POP with persistent or extensive vaginal erosions.

- Radiation to the pelvic cavity.

- Vagina and its outlet (hiatus) are so dilated (enlarged) that the pessary will not stay in position.

The following are additional tips that may be helpful to know about the use of a pessary:

- Intercourse is possible with certain kinds of pessaries in place. Check with your physician to see if the pessary you will be using will interfere and need to be removed prior to intercourse. Some women find it uncomfortable to have sex with their pessary in. Some men find it enhances sensation for them, while others find it uncomfortable. If you have a pessary that can be left in during intercourse, you will have to experiment to see how it will work for you as a couple.

- A pessary may pop out when you bear down to have a bowel movement. It is helpful to bridge the labia (hold your 1st and 2nd fingers in a V position and push them up against the vaginal lips while having a bowel movement).

- The vagina is a closed canal; the pessary cannot shift or get lost anywhere else inside of the body. It can pop out of the vagina if the pessary is too small. If it pops out without bearing down, contact your physician; you likely need a different size or type.

- A pessary will very rarely set off a metal detector at an airport if there are metal components in it (few have metal). Ask the clinician fitting your pessary whether yours has metal and if so, remove it and use an over-the-counter disposable pessary while traveling by plane.

- A pessary may need to be resized with weight gain or loss. A pessary will typically last two to three years before replacement is needed.

- Some patients who use pessaries over an extended period may find it necessary to switch to a smaller size. Some research indicates that POP status may improve over time with extended pessary use.

- Pessaries may be beneficial for elderly patients with POP who are not candidates for surgery because of compromised health. These women will typically need their physicians to remove, clean, and reinsert the pessary.

- Patients that can't be fitted for a pessary, feel uncomfortable with a pessary in, or have problems with a pessary popping out are potential candidates for surgery.

- Women with severe POP that are advised against having surgery or who don't want to go through surgery may be able to use two ring pessaries together for additional support.

Pessaries play a significant role in POP treatment for temporary control of symptoms and for permanent use in those women who cannot or do not want to have surgery. No matter what type or grade of POP you have, there is a strong possibility that at some point you will be introduced to the use of a pessary.

It is relatively common for women who start POP treatment utilizing a pessary to shift to surgery in time. We live in an extremely active society, and although pessaries are relatively easy to use, busy women often prefer a more maintenance-free solution.

Impressa

Impressa is a single use over-the-counter tampon-like, disposable pessary designed to temporarily prevent stress urinary incontinence. While this non-absorbent, disposable product is designed for incontinence, it may also have value for women in early stages of POP by providing internal support during activities that create pressure on the pelvic floor, such as fitness activities. It can also come in handy for flight travel in place of a traditional pessary to avoid concerns about security screening setting off alarms with the few pessaries that do contain metal.

Kegel Exercises

Let's review some basics to clarify the source of the pelvic floor issues women commonly navigate. The pelvic organs (bladder, uterus, and rectum) are supported from below by the levator ani muscles, also known as the PC muscles or the pelvic floor muscle group. The PC below along with ligaments suspending organs from above provide support and stabilize organs in the pelvic cavity. The bowl-shaped PC muscle has 3 individual arms which can become weakened or damaged as a result of childbirth, menopause, and/or lifestyle, behaviors, or co-existing health conditions. Multiple structures that enable urination, defecation, and sexual function pass through this muscle structure, and that is where aspects of women's vaginal and pelvic wellness start to break down, literally.

Kegel exercises were developed in 1948 by Dr. Arnold Kegel and are beneficial for nearly all women to optimize pelvic floor health, as well as have value for post-surgical pelvic floor strength and maintenance. Dr. Kegel was light years ahead of his peers, recognizing the significance of strengthening the PC muscle. Kegels should not be viewed as a "quick-fix" for prolapse, however they should be utilized for life-long maintenance of PC muscle strength much like brushing your teeth maintains oral health. If practiced prior to and throughout pregnancy (check with your physician first, particularly if you have miscarriage concerns), the pelvic floor remains more elastic and resistant to damage during childbirth. If practiced following childbirth, Kegels may restore a degree of tone to the muscles of the pelvic floor. Kegel exercises can be performed anywhere in multiple positions, lying down, sitting, or standing, although when first learning proper Kegel technique, it is best to perform them lying down until familiar with PC contraction sensation and proper form.

A Kegel muscle contraction is the same contraction that occurs to stop the flow of urine. It can be helpful to establish a ritual time and place to perform Kegel exercises. While you will achieve the strongest contraction while lying down, there is value in building up PC integrity while sitting or standing to optimize PC muscle tissue fibers from multiple angles of contraction as well as contracting against gravity.

PC strength will fluctuate from day to day based on many factors including your general health, diet-related bloating, or abdominal distention related to rectocele-generated gas. Muscle has memory; it is imperative to stay the course during the first 12 weeks of any program regardless how bloated you are feeling. Establishing a Kegel exercise habit as part of your daily rituals is of value to maintain life-long continence and sexual sensation along with reducing POP symptoms. The PC contraction will feel stronger on days you are not bloated, but even on days you feel bloated and the contraction feels weak, you can continue to improve baseline strength.

Women with a higher grade of POP severity (grades 3 or 4) might not be able to contract the PC deeply or maintain a Kegel contraction. It is also important to note that some women have tight pelvic floor muscles. It is important for this sector to capture guidance from a physical therapist regarding how to Kegel; they are the experts in the pelvic floor muscle and soft tissue structures. A PT can help women understand the difference between the PC muscle contracting in and up which stops the flow of urine, as opposed to a Valsalva maneuver which pushes vaginal tissues down and out.

A Kegel contraction does not tighten the abdominal, buttock, or thigh muscles. The PC contraction is specific to the levator ani muscles supporting internal organs. It is of value to keep other muscles relaxed when doing Kegels. Place a hand on your belly to detect unintentional abdominal action (there may be some minimal ab contraction, but do not intentionally contract the abs when doing a Kegel).

To initially locate the PC muscle contraction, insert one or two fingers into the vagina (wash hands first please!) and squeeze your PC muscle until you can feel the contraction around your fingers. If not sure how contracting the PC muscle feels, sit on the toilet to urinate, and then stop the flow of urine mid-stream (once only ladies to recognize the contraction, not repetitively). Another method is to contract the way you would if you were attempting to avoid passing gas.

Once a woman is able to effectively contract the PC, she can contract it randomly (but not continuously) throughout the day to strengthen her pelvic floor as well as to protect it prior to lifting anything heavy including children. The more routinely contracting the PC prior to heavy lifting is practiced, the more likely it is to become habit, particularly valuable to women with babies and toddlers.

Advantageous times to practice a few Kegels are while cooking, using your phone, brushing your teeth, standing in line at the store, or while watching TV (kegel throughout the commercials). There are conflicting schools of thought regarding value of Kegel contractions when in a sitting position; I find this position a valuable variation because I spend so much time on the computer and alternating positions target muscle tissue differently. Once your pattern is established, it will become second nature to spontaneously contract without thought. Whether nonsurgical or surgical treatments are used to treat POP, it is a good idea to continue to practice Kegel exercises to maintain the habit. Kegels can and should be practiced by all adult women - there is no such thing as too old to Kegel.

Doing multiple sets of Kegels is often recommended by clinicians but may over-fatigue the pelvic floor. A single set of 10 contractions completed correctly with proper form, holding the contraction longer, and attempting to contract more deeply, has greater value. Quality over quantity.

Individuals who want to take kegeling to the next level can incorporate Kegel breathing into their daily ritual. To Kegel breathe, a meditative practice that may also help you relax while strengthening your pelvic floor, relax your belly as you breath in and as you slowly let the air out, contract your PC muscle and hold the contraction for as long as possible. This can be done any time throughout the day. Kegel breathe randomly throughout the day rather than repetitiously in a single session. The idea is to "wake up" and strengthen your PC, not gridlock it into a nonfunctional painfully locked, tight pelvic floor.

PC Strengthening Devices

I have experienced multiple unnerving women's health symptoms at this point in my life. Urine retention. Stress urinary incontinence. Overactive bladder. Chronic constipation. A frustrating episode of fecal incontinence at the airport prior to heading off to Nepal related to my nonprofit efforts. While I never felt highly stigmatized by these experiences, I had never given much thought to talking out loud about them prior to becoming a POP patient advocate and realizing how incapacitating the shroud of silence is to women's health awareness.

One of the perks of being a vocal POP advocate is I am approached from time to time to test nonsurgical programs, treatments, and devices developed to address a weak pelvic floor and/or accompanying symptoms. I nearly always enthusiastically agree to play guinea pig. My intent is to evaluate new tools developed to strengthen and optimize pelvic floor strength and function to both enable me to share insights with women experiencing POP, but also to augment my personal POP "maintenance for life" ritual. I have a drawer full of devices I have tested over the years.

There is a variety of medical devices available to help strengthen the PC muscle, such as wired wearables, pad wearables, vaginally insertable app-based devices with probes in many shapes and sizes, electrical stimulus and pressure sensitive devices, and non-app insertable vaginal cones, weights, or ceramic eggs which a PC contraction holds in place to provide weighted resistance for a period of time while standing or walking. Some app-based devices provide biofeedback to enable the user to visualize contraction strength. These devices/programs are designed to be inserted only during the training cycle, typically between 5-30 minutes. I've tried multiple PC strengthening devices over the years and as a woman post-surgery, I've found the devices most user-friendly are those which are relatively compact, provide biofeedback to enable user to literally "see" the contraction, and clean up easily which makes them convenient for travel.

My current favorite device is Leva, a biofeedback app-based pelvic floor strengthening tool. For a decade post-surgery in 2008, I had no leakage issues; my transvaginal POP and sling repairs held strong. But as often occurs with time, age and lifestyle impacted my pelvic floor ballast. Despite my successful surgical repairs and a decades-long pelvic floor and core fitness regimen, I started experiencing minor urinary incontinence issues. Gastroesophageal reflux disease (GERD) became a facet of daily navigation and included a persistent, aggressive cough which most certainly trashed my pelvic floor integrity. When I coughed, I could place my hand on the tissues surrounding the introitus (the vaginal opening), and literally feel them blasting downward every time my GERD hack occurred.

Leva is a Food and Drug Administration (FDA) cleared pelvic floor muscle trainer with visible biofeedback technology that enables patients to view the "contraction in action" in real-time on their cell phones. The developer's intent is to target the muscles predominately responsible for maintaining continence by rehabilitating and strengthening weak pelvic floor muscles to treat stress, mixed, and mild to moderate urge incontinence in women, including overactive bladder. Patients can complete training in the privacy of their homes in 5 minutes per day. The treatment is performed in a gravity-feed standing position, unique from any other device available at the time of testing. This device enables patients to track, review, and share their data with clinicians (Leva is prescribed for patients by physicians).

What I discovered in the first 2 weeks of training truly surprised me. Turns out I had developed a habit of keeping both core and floor muscles simultaneously contracted nearly all the time in an attempt to maintain core/floor strength. I did not recognize that I was walking around in a state of pelvic floor lockdown, reducing my pelvic floor strength (to be fully functional, it is pivotal to fully relax pelvic floor muscles prior to contracting them, which Leva instructs you to do during the exercising phase). Interestingly, I quickly recognized a reduction in overactive bladder urge once I learned to fully relax my pelvic floor, and leakage was radically reduced so quickly it was shocking. Another quick perk was urine hesitancy also quickly fell by the wayside. I did not realize the daily habits I had established were disabling rather than helping my pelvic floor health. As I relaxed into the program, contracting the core and floor as well as rectal and urinary sphincters separately became easy-peasy. While intent of testing Leva was related to urinary incontinence, I was curious if there would be additional value regarding other pelvic floor related issues. There was. The concerns I wanted to address:

- Minor urine leakage when I coughed or sneezed.

- Minor urine leakage sitting up to get out of bed in the morning.

- High stress days = overactive bladder running amuck.

- Weak urine stream.

- Urinary hesitancy.

- Loss of sensation in anal sphincter.

- Fecal urgency.

Improvements:

- Stronger urine stream.

- Could relax pelvic floor completely.

- Reduced cough/sneeze leakage.

- Less frequent leakage getting out of bed.

- No urination hesitancy.

- Could relax pelvic floor completely.

- Improved ability to contract core/floor as separate units.

- Much more cognizant of body tensing (in all areas, not just the pelvic floor).

- Radical reduction in OAB symptoms.

- Anal sensation and contraction improved; no longer needed to run to assure getting to the bathroom in time.

As I moved further into my test period, not only did bladder issues and symptoms continue to improve, but Leva biofeedback additionally helped me understand the live action state of my core and pelvic floor, as well as how I reacted to external or internal stimuli. I no longer needed to make 2 bathroom stops during 3-hour road trips; I rarely need to stop at all. Daily bathroom runs radically reduced in number, and instead of getting up 3 times a night to pee, 1 overnight trip did the trick. The repetitive urinary urge when working at my desk for long hours stopped. When I decide to take a break and get up after several hours at the keyboard, I recognize that I have the urge to pee, but I can walk to the bathroom; no need to rush. And most significantly, Leva not only helped me recognize I had a tight pelvic floor, the protocol also helped me understand how to completely relax my pelvic floor muscles prior to a contraction. There is no other device I have tested that effectively included this step in their program. The live-action visual Leva provides on the app to both relax and contract the pelvic floor is priceless; it is doubtful the end result would have been as optimized without it.

I find it questionable that any woman's pelvic floor strength is top-notch every single day. I could see as well as feel my pelvic floor strength increasing week by week. Numbers don't lie. While I wandered into the program with what I thought was a fairly strong pelvic floor, I recognized that despite having a strong base knowledge of what the PC muscle is and does, I was making several mistakes in my strengthening program. What I found particularly priceless was the days I didn't do well on the numerical scale, the program validated how I felt physically.

Many women newly diagnosed with pelvic organ prolapse are not yet ready to jump to the page of surgery, and that is a good thing. It is beneficial for women to understand vaginal and pelvic floor health and maintenance basics prior to taking the leap. We are creatures of habit with hectic lifestyles and rarely recognize poor pelvic floor habits unless we are informed by a clinician after the damage is done. Our routines enable us to navigate our day-to-day craziness, subconsciously committing us to rituals that frame nearly every waking and many of our sleeping hours.

It is imperative women educate themselves about their female anatomy. Women must understand the value of both strengthening and relaxing the pelvic floor and experiment with diverse nonsurgical treatments until they find the right fit for their needs. If/when women move forward with surgery, maintaining pelvic floor muscle function is critical to optimize pelvic and pelvic floor health long term. Why wouldn't we want to maintain the integrity of our urinary, defecatory, and sexual health systems?

Pelvic Floor And Core Exercise Programs

It is critical women are advised to optimize pelvic floor health during women's wellness exams. It's beneficial prior to pregnancy; a healthy pelvic floor may increase the potential for more flexible tissue, an easier delivery, and speedier recovery. It's beneficial post-partum to recover former pelvic floor muscle tone to reduce the risk of POP progression. It's beneficial post hysterectomy and POP surgery to maintain the benefit of repairs. As women, we must recognize the value of pulling our core in and our pelvic floor up randomly throughout the day to maintain muscle tone.

There are many exercise regimens available for pelvic floor strengthening. An exercise regimen is only beneficial if it is one you will continue to utilize. Some women prefer a condensed program because they have little free time; others prefer a diverse, detailed format. The regimen that worked for me was taking the specific exercises that worked well for my body from different programs and modifying the exercise routine I already had in place.

Pay attention to the impact a regimen has on all areas of your body rather than just the pelvic floor. If you feel a program is causing pain or problems anywhere in your body, it probably is. Back or knee pain are indicators that the program might not be appropriate for you. The same can be said for programs or particular core or floor exercises that increase vaginal or rectal pressure. There are multiple appropriate core and floor exercise programs available online; some are fee-based apps, some are free. POP programs should specifically mention they are related to addressing pelvic organ prolapse or urinary incontinence.

Hormone Replacement Therapy

Menopause is the 2nd leading cause of pelvic organ prolapse. Pain with intimacy, a relatively common POP symptom, all too often is the consequence of estrogen loss related during perimenopause or menopause, resulting in atrophied, irritated tissues. While the emotional distress women experience regarding organs and tissues peeking out of the vagina during sex-play may hinder engagement, pain with intimacy can shut the door completely.

Beyond the loss of muscle tissue strength and elasticity, estrogen depletion may result in vaginal and vulval tissue becoming irritated, thin, dry, and less supple.

Vaginal secretions are reduced, resulting in decreased lubrication during sex. Dry, itchy, fragile vulvovaginal tissues are susceptible to injury, tearing, and bleeding during intercourse. Intimacy may become so painful that sex stops occurring at all. When a woman does not engage in intercourse regularly during and following menopause, the vagina may become shorter and/or narrower, an additional cause of pain when intercourse is attempted, even when using a lubricant. Atrophy can be a considerable roadblock for women already struggling with POP-related self-esteem issues. The impact to sexual satisfaction and relationships can be devastating.

Michael Goodman, MD, a world-renowned menopause and sexual medicine specialist as well as a cosmetic gynecologist, has spent decades providing innovative and integrative women's healthcare. As a surgeon, teacher, author, and menopause expert, he shines a light to clarify reality vs. misconception regarding hormone depletion. A phone call to Dr. Goodman quickly shifted from a casual conversation into a valuable class in hormone therapy.

· · · ● · ● · ● · ·

Q. WOMEN OFTEN FEAR TRADITIONAL HORMONE REPLACE-MENT THERAPY (HRT). CAN YOU CLARIFY THE DIFFERENCE BETWEEN HRT AND BIOIDENTICAL HORMONE REPLACEMENT THERAPY?

The difference between bioidentical hormone replacement therapy (BHRT) and hormone replacement therapy (HRT) is often misinterpreted, so let's begin by clarifying the difference between BHRT, HRT, and compounded hormones.

There are 3 types of estrogen in women, estriol (E3), estradiol (E2), and estrone (E1). Estradiol is the most commonly used estrogen in hormone replacement therapy. Estradiol can be considered the "natural" replacement since it is the estrogen in women's ovulatory follicles the ovaries used to produce prior to menopause. Estrogen is available in pill, patch, oil, suppository, gel, injection, vaginally inserted ring form, or by means of oral or transdermal (absorbed into the body through the skin) transfer. Estrone is the riskiest estrogen related to the breast tissue, and estriol is the estrogen produced by the placenta in pregnant women, not by the ovary.

Estrogen, progesterone, and testosterone are isomers (compounds with an identical chemical formula), structures that may be synthesized in the lab by splitting off side-chains from "plant sterols" such as wild Mexican yams or soybeans to produce the biologically or molecularly identical compounds used in the so-called bioidenticals. The hormone Premarin, which until the past 10 years was the most commonly prescribed hormone replacement, can be considered "natural" as it is directly produced from a "natural" source (pregnant mares' urine), which contains 10 different estrogenic compounds. BHRT by definition is not truly "natural" (coming directly from a plant or animal source) but is derived from a natural source. Since yams, soybeans, and horse urine are all plant/animal sourced, they all technically fit into the "bioidentical" format. However, what is of significance is how precisely and appropriately they are utilized within the body to generate the most benefit with minimal to no side effects.

Compounding hormones is a blending of different kinds of hormones into a variety of dosages and dosage forms, creating multiple options to provide a more targeted benefit to suit women's individual needs, such as combining E2, progesterone, testosterone, and perhaps others into a single application product. Compounded hormones are usually less expensive if you do not have insurance covering these types of hormone replacement therapies. Compounded formulations do not undergo the strict manufacturing and purity standards testing that their FDA-approved counterparts such as Premarin do. However, despite this unregulated environment, compounded hormones are widely popular with patients seeking more "personalized" medicine.

Interestingly, all of the estradiol (E2) in the world to my knowledge, comes from one of two companies in Germany, Mallinckrodt Pharmaceuticals or Organon Pharmaceuticals. These compounds are either sold to Pharma, who make such products as Vivelle Dot, Climara patch, DiviGel, Estrace (estradiol tablets) etc. or sold to wholesalers, who sell directly to compounding pharmacies. They all can be considered "BHRT".

So... while the term "BHRT" usually refers to the compounded product, in truth there are two types of bioidenticals, "FDA-Approved" (which have been tested for purity and concentration) and "compounded bioidenticals" which are not. While both are inherently safe, especially if you know and trust the compounder, commercial bioidenticals are inherently safer than the compounded ones, as they have been FDA tested and received approval. Compounded bioidenticals are what is called "off-label;" traditionally utilized for a specific purpose but not officially approved for usage. As dosing and application sites have not been standardized, and as many clinicians use robust (compounded) dosing, BHRT must be considered less safe than so-called "traditional HRT." Thus, it is imperative that, if compounded BHRT is used, the specific practitioner prescribing should be researched. I would hope the provider is a gynecologist or a hormonal medicine specialist and not a med-spa provid er.

Q. PLEASE DISTINGUISH THE DIFFERENCE BETWEEN LUBRICAT-ING GELS AND CREAMS VS. HORMONE REPLACEMENT THERAPY TO REPLENISH VAGINAL MOISTURE.

Lubricating gels and creams lubricate. Vaginal HRT, whether estradiol, estriol, DHEA, or testosterone, nourish, normalize, and regenerate the vaginal skin to be able to stretch better and self-lubricate without burning or tearing.

Q. IS THERE ANY BENEFIT TO INTRODUCING LOW-DOSE ESTRO-GEN THERAPY EARLY TO PREVENT OR REDUCE ATROPHY?

There is a huge benefit to this. As my grandma used to say, "an ounce of prevention is worth a pound of cure". Local vaginal and perineal HT containing microdoses of any of the above hormones (question 2) singularly or in combination is both wildly successful and not considered traditional systemic HT. The doses of vulvovaginal therapy contain per week the same amount or hormone exposure as HRT or BHRT does per day.

Q. CAN YOU SPEAK TO "SHRINKAGE" OF VAGINAL LENGTH, WIDTH, AND THE VAGINAL OPENING THAT OCCURS WITH ATRO-PHY?

It is a "use it or lose it" phenomenon. When hormonal levels dive, the vaginal cells receive no nutrition and shrink or die, leading to what the question describes. Again, "...ounce of prevention..." The "cure..." takes time but is usually fully successful, and consists of first developing vaginal health, then slowly dilating the vaginal length and caliber with progressive dilator therapy. This timetable may be shortened with the use of an EBD (Energy-Based Device) such as laser or radiofrequency (RF) treatments.

Q. IS VAGINAL DILATOR USE OF VALUE TO TREAT ATROPHY, AND IF SO, HOW SHOULD IT BE USED, AND WHEN IS IT INTRODUCED?

Yes, effective. Use begins after the vagina and vulvar vestibule is well estrogenized, which usually takes ~ 6 months with HT, or ~ 3 months with laser + HT. In dilator therapy, cone-shaped, usually rigid plastic or hard rubber cones of progressively increasing length and/or caliber are utilized until the vagina is of sufficient caliber and length to accommodate enjoyable vaginal intercourse.

Q. WHAT IS YOUR OPINION OF THE USE OF BIOIDENTICAL HORMONES VS. LASER OR RADIO FREQUENCY TO TREAT VAGINAL ATROPHY?

They both work and are viable options. As I wrote above, using vaginal micro dose hormone therapy is effective in more than 90% of patients, but takes a while. Use of laser or RF, especially if either micro dose E2 or E3 or DHEA is utilized after therapy, will speed up the process by 50%. But it will cost you $2500-$3000 and is not covered by insurance.

Q. CLEARLY MENOPAUSE IS NOT THE ONLY CAUSE OF REDUCED ESTROGEN LEVELS. CAN YOU CLARIFY OTHER POSSIBLE CONDITIONS AND CAUSES, PARTICULARLY THOSE THAT MAY OCCUR IN WOMEN UNDER 50?

The most likely cause of reduced estrogen levels in women under 50 is of course the lowering estradiol levels that occur with ovarian aging and loss of ovulatory follicles, as 50% of women go through menopause prior to age 50. Of course, any therapy, surgical, radiological or chemotherapy, that removes or eliminates ovarian function will cause estrogen levels to jump off the pier. Hysterectomy that removes ovaries results in immediate cessation of E2 levels. Smokers and diabetics lose ovarian function earlier. Liver disease may also alter estrogen levels.

Q. IN APOPS SPACE, AT THE 6 WEEK POINT POST-SURGERY IF A WOMAN IS STILL EXPERIENCING PAIN, THE FIRST THING SHE IS CONCERNED ABOUT IS SURGICAL COMPLICATIONS. CAN YOU CLARIFY WHETHER ATROPHY NOT HAVING BEEN ADDRESSED PRIOR TO POP SURGERY COULD BE A POSSIBLE SOURCE OF POST-SURGICAL PAIN, AND SHARE YOUR OPINION REGARDING THE USE OF VAGINAL ESTROGEN PRE AND POST-SURGERY AS AN ADJUNCT THERAPY FOR POST-SURGICAL VAGINAL HEALING?

I reconstruct and rebuild vaginal floors. I work in exactly the same space as urogynecologists. It is rare that vaginal reconstructive surgery is an emergency or must be performed ASAP. It is my conviction, based on both clinical and histological data that a healthy, well-estrogenized vagina will heal far better than an atrophic one, so if I am to operate on a peri/post-menopausal woman with vulvovaginal atrophy, I require a minimum of 3 months of vaginal therapy prior to surgery, and continuation of this therapy beginning 1 month after surgery. Simply put, a well-estrogenized vagina and vulvar vestibule is a healthy vagina and vulvar vestibule and will heal earlier and better.

· · · · **·** · **·** · · · ·

Hormone replacement may also be of value in conjunction with other treatments. Although hormone replacement therapy alone will not be of huge benefit for women with advanced POP, it can be helpful for women experiencing low hormone levels who are in early stages of POP. Most women who have experienced or are in treatment for cancer will not be able to utilize this treatment option, so it is important the clinician providing hormone therapy is aware of previous or current cancer treatment.

Nonsurgical Vaginal Rejuvenation

The term vaginal rejuvenation can be a bit confusing since there are both surgical and nonsurgical vaginal rejuvenation procedures available. Heat-based nonsurgical radio frequency or laser treatments were initially developed to address incontinence and atrophy. Nonsurgical vaginal rejuvenation should be more appropriately named vaginal tissue regeneration since these heat-producing procedures literally produce new collagen and elastin within the vaginal wall tissue. Heat-based nonsurgical vaginal rejuvenation treatments have been studied in Europe since 2008 and are readily available around the world at this point.

Nonsurgical vaginal rejuvenation procedures provide temporary improvement of symptoms being addressed. Vaginal rejuvenation surgical procedures such as labiaplasty, vaginoplasty, and perineoplasty are permanent repairs that address damage related to childbirth or the aesthetic vaginal, labial, or perineum concerns which women are born with that cause discomfort or concern.

Nonsurgical vaginal rejuvenation may be of value to reduce the severity of some symptoms of pelvic organ prolapse. Radiofrequency projects heat deep into tissues, improving tissue structural integrity; laser treatment makes microscopic perforations in vaginal tissue, generating a wound/healing process. These therapies strengthen mucosal tissues (the lining in your vagina and rectum) by stimulating production of collagen and elastin, important connective structural tissue. While heat-based vaginal rejuvenation is not FDA-approved for all vaginal treatment uses, research has documented benefits such as a reduction in incontinence (stress, urge), overactive bladder symptoms, and possibly some benefit for fecal incontinence, as well as reduced vaginal atrophy (dryness). Additional benefits that may occur are a temporary tightening of the vaginal space (less vaginal space could improve organ support) and increased intimate sensation. Research additionally indicates these treatments are of value for tightening external labial lip tissue sag for those interested in the aesthetic value.

There will undoubtedly be considerably more validated research related to these treatments, both solo and in combination with other treatments, over the next several years. At the current time, insurance generally does not cover vaginal rejuvenation procedures, so treatment can be cost-prohibitive. While nonsurgical vaginal rejuvenation therapies do not permanently fix POP, they may reduce symptoms.

Women of childbearing age should have a negative pregnancy test prior to receiving these therapies, as well as a recent pelvic exam and a few years of normal Pap smears (cervix cell scraping to test for cancer). While dermatologists and plastic surgeons and even med-spas may provide these treatments, it is best to access those provided by a gynecologist, urogynecologist, or a cosmetic gynecologist since these are the women's health providers most familiar with vaginal health conditions. Safety first!

Treatments typically take place every 4-6 weeks for the series of three treatments in year one, followed by annual maintenance. Information women should share with clinicians prior to treatment is intrauterine device (IUD) use, implanted Interstim device, herpes or other sexually transmitted conditions, implanted mesh related to pelvic organ prolapse or incontinence surgery (radio frequency is appropriate for patients with mesh, laser is not), mesh complications, chronic vaginal or pelvic pain, or pregnancy. Fully inform your practitioner of all vaginal health concerns.

Women experiencing atrophy related to cancer therapies may find these treatments a beneficial alternative to the hormone treatments that may be a cancer conflict and no longer utilized. Treatments are typically avoided in women actively undergoing treatment for cancer but may be used in some women post-cancer treatment at the discretion of their practitioners.

Vaginal and pelvic health ballast shifts continuously for women throughout the life cycle. Like most women, my body gets a bit sassy from time to time. It is important women educate themselves about diverse POP treatment options prior to deciding which will be the best to fit their needs.

Several years ago, despite having effectively balanced my hormones with prescribed bioidenticals for 20+ years, I was a bit disillusioned that I couldn't seem
to get the atrophy under control despite modifying my regimen. Time for the
big guns. I decided to explore nonsurgical vaginal rejuvenation therapy myself to
better understand the treatment and value.

I reviewed multiple vaginal tissue restoration research papers and engaged in conversations with a few companies that provide these services, as well as physicians
who utilized them. To say I wanted more information is an understatement. I had
the opportunity to sit in on a radio frequency treatment provided to a patient
during a physician training course, and as a patient advocate was able to question
her immediately following the session. My next step was coordinating schedules
to jump on the table to experiment with radio frequency up close and personal
at a gynecologist's office. A nurse practitioner provided the treatments, as well as
shared valuable insights during the treatment process. The following information
is a blend of feedback provided by several gynecologists and urogynecologists
regarding both types of heat-based procedures.

· · · · · ● · ● · · ·

Q. WHO CAN PROVIDE THERMIVA RADIOFREQUENCY TREAT-
MENTS?

*While many in plastic surgery and aesthetics are advancing their knowledge and
skillset in vaginal restoration procedures, it makes sense for women with pelvic
organ prolapse to locate a gynecologist or other clinician who specializes in women's
pelvic health to provide this procedure if possible. POP is complicated and you want
someone who is very familiar with female anatomy providing these kinds of pelvic
procedures - whether radio frequency or laser. Multiple conditions can exist at the
same time in a woman's pelvic zone.*

Q. HOW DO THESE TREATMENTS WORK?

*Heat is the source of these treatments; radio frequency generates heat, laser therapy
creates thousands of tiny, deep perforations in tissue to generate a healing response.
Both kinds of treatments stimulate collagen and elastin production which strength-
ens tissues in the vaginal canal. Explore how many treatments your clinician has
provided - you want someone with experience. Too much heat in one area during
a laser procedure may cause blistering-this can cause some temporary discomfort.*

However, both treatment types are considered very safe procedures.

Q. WHAT DO THE TREATMENTS COST?

Cost varies significantly from clinician to clinician with both of these procedures, from a few hundred dollars per procedure to a few thousand. The individual medical practice sets the price; it tends to be more expensive on the coasts compared to the Midwest.

Q. WHAT IF I'VE HAD MESH SURGERY?

Use of laser in women who have mesh, IUD, any kind of internal devices is not validated by research at this stage. Radiofrequency generates less heat, which is more appropriate for use in women with mesh. As always, take your questions to your consultation and reveal all devices and procedures you've had to your clinician for the best outcome.

Q. CAN THESE TREATMENTS BE OF VALUE FOR OTHER CONDITIONS BESIDES PELVIC ORGAN PROLAPSE OR INCONTINENCE?

These treatments may be worth exploring for treatment of Lichen Sclerosis and Ehlers-Danlos syndrome. The benefits for these conditions have been minimally explored in Europe and show promise. It will take time to capture data.

Q. WILL I NEED MORE THAN ONE TREATMENT?

Both laser and radiofrequency treatments require three treatments the first year, with an annual treatment suggested after that to maintain. Women may be happy with results after the first treatment and cancel the others. This is not a good idea for long-term value. There will be swelling from first treatment which can simulate success, but it takes 3 treatments to properly jumpstart collagen-building process, which is what brings results that continue over the next year related to the symptom(s) being treated. Long-term results are currently unknown and are believed to start to fade about a year post-treatment, thus the annual reboot.

Q. DO I NEED TO CONTINUE MY CORE/FLOOR EXERCISES IF I HAVE A VAGINAL RESTORATION PROCEDURE?

It is important women recognize engaging in additional forms of maintenance (pelvic floor and core strengthening) prior to and post treatments will bring them the greatest value in achieving and maintaining results. It is important to remain proactive with pelvic health in general and pelvic floor muscle integrity in the long run, whether utilizing nonsurgical or surgical treatments.

Q. WILL RESULTS BE DIFFERENT FOR A WOMAN IN HER 40'S THAN A WOMAN IN HER 60S?

Results are reported to be similar regardless the age of a woman. However, length of time to achieve these results during active treatment may vary a bit. Success is based on patient feedback; results are related to quality-of-life impact. While there are studies to validate tissue regeneration, there is no standardized test analyzing vaginal tissue post-procedure. If the patient recognizes she has less incontinence, or discomfort from atrophy, or sensation is increased, the procedure has done what it is supposed to do. Impact on a patient's quality of life is the target.

Q. DO I NEED TO HAVE ANY TESTS PRIOR TO THE TREATMENT?

A pelvic exam is required prior to the procedure to ensure an undiagnosed condition or health concern does not exist. This can be provided by your gynecologist or primary health clinician. On-site treatment evaluation should also include info about other pelvic surgeries you've had which may disclose concerns (for example, complications from hysterectomy or bowel resection that may cause organ shift or have created excessive scar tissue, or the patient has considerable undiagnosed pain). It may be necessary to go through other treatments such as estrogen therapy or dilators to balance your pelvic tissue health prior to moving forward with vaginal tissue restoration. These treatments are not a miracle cure to fix all vaginal health conditions.

Q. WILL THESE TREATMENTS FIX FAILED POP SURGERY?

Vaginal restoration procedures will not address prior POP surgical failure related to incompetent surgeon or complications beyond the surgeon's control. These procedures may have some value however related to longer success of mesh-free surgeries or age and/or menopause-related vaginal health concerns. Multiple aspects of these procedures are uncertain because women have multiple lifestyle, behavioral, and coexisting condition POP causal factors.

Q. WILL THERE BE ANY DISCOMFORT WITH MY PROCEDURE?

Typically, there is very little discomfort, if any. Some women may experience warmth or redness, and some women may have a little vaginal discharge or bleeding after treatment.

Q. DO I NEED TO COMPLETELY SHAVE MY PUBIC AREA BEFORE TREATMENT?

Shaving or closely trimming the hair in the pubic area is recommended; this is for better contact with the skin to achieve therapeutic temperatures.

• • • ● • ● • ● • •

I shared information about my personal exploration with radiofrequency from November 2016 through January 2017 in APOPS website articles in a series of 4 posts. Here's an instant replay of my final evaluation.

VAGINAL TISSUE REGENERATION THERAPY PART 4: NEXT STEPS

When new health therapies appear in the relatively young medical specialty field of pelvic organ prolapse (POP), especially when they sound too good to be true, we tend to dismiss them as snake-oil quackery. While research in vaginal tissue regeneration therapy (more commonly known as vaginal rejuvenation therapy) has progressed considerably over the past 15 years validating the benefits of treatment for atrophy and incontinence, some clinicians and patients remain skeptical and consider them cosmetic at best. Based on personal experience, I can assure those who have yet to recognize the value of these temporary treatments to move forward with an open mind. There is indeed a potential benefit to women experiencing a loss of QOL related to symptoms POP exhibits.

Women have many options to address the symptoms of POP, including surgery, lasers, radio frequency, systemic or topical estrogen therapy to reboot lubrication, biofeedback, or e-stim (both in-office procedures and over-the-counter devices are available), and obviously, Kegels or pelvic floor/core exercise regimens. At-home therapies should be utilized routinely to maintain the long-term benefit of surgery, and of course are a pivotal pelvic health maintenance tool whether opting for surgery or not. Vaginal rejuvenation therapy typically needs to be minimally rebooted annually. The theory behind these treatments is heat regenerates collagen and elastin, to return vaginal tissues to a healthy strong, plump, and moist state.

I was skeptical and pensive at the onset of my exploration, capturing info slowly from European studies, US-based studies, webinars, attendance at live procedures, then moving forward to personally test the waters. There are 2 types of tooling for nonsurgical vaginal rejuvenation treatments, laser and radio frequency, including a combo of them used together, the difference being the depth of penetration and degree of heat generation. I initially chose to experiment with lower heat radio frequency because I have transvaginal mesh inserted for cystocele and rectocele repairs.

To say I was both shocked and pleased at the result of my treatments is an understatement. There is zero doubt that this therapy has considerable value as a treatment for many of the symptoms of POP. Are there concerns to address? Absolutely. Cost, availability, long-term efficacy, and long-term impact on soft tissue need to be evaluated. We have much more to research and much more to validate before nonsurgical rejuvenation is approved by Medicare, the mothership of insurance coverage. But there is zero doubt in my mind we absolutely should push the protocol forward.

As of 2022, I am 14+ years past successful transvaginal mesh surgery. I personally have not found a single minimally invasive treatment that comes close to reducing numerous overlapping POP symptoms (or those that come post-surgery as a result of the aging process) that improve QOL the way vaginal rejuvenation therapy does, and I have experimented with multiple types of nonsurgical treatments and over the counter devices above and beyond having had POP surgery. I have a drawer full of tools and devices that could undoubtedly make a grown man blush, exploring in an extensive quest to share information with APOPS patient following. Placebo effect has no impact on me (decades of navigating MS have made me acutely aware of sensation and lack of sensation regardless of where it occurs in my body). Playing guinea pig enables me to better recognize tools that are of value, and I do my best to share the information I capture in an unbiased way with the women APOPS serves.

The best way I can explain the profound shift I experienced with vaginal rejuvenation therapy is it felt like a complete reboot of internal pelvic and vaginal tissue support. My guts hadn't felt this great since I was in my early 30's prior to my pregnancy.

The upside:

- Overactive bladder sensation was gone.

- No leaks when I sneezed or coughed.

- No need to zoom to the bathroom when urge to defecate occurred.

- Pelvic, vaginal, and rectal pressure disappeared.

- Atrophy was no longer an issue.

- Urine stream was strong.

- Stool was normal shape and size.

- Only 1 trip to the bathroom in overnight hours.

The downside:

- These amazing changes began to diminish at 3 months, and by 4 months were gone.

- As the symptoms I struggled with prior to my treatments returned, I found them annoyingly worse than they made me feel prior to treatment - obviously because I felt so great when my tissue quality was optimized.

With vaginal rejuvenation therapy, I literally experienced how great my pelvic floor and contents could feel again.

My exploration convinced me how valuable these new treatments are to address multiple common POP QOL symptoms. Women with POP know the mantra, pull your floor up, hold your core in. But the reality is despite pulling things up and in, despite doing "all the right stuff", despite having successful POP surgery and moving forward with our lives, the aging process can generate some issues that impact our comfort, our sexuality, our self-esteem, and our general QOL.

My final RF treatment took place in January 2017. Post RF treatment, my pelvic and vaginal spaces felt the best they had felt in decades. Pressure sensations were gone. My urinary and defecatory compartments worked great.

Do I want to "recapture my recharged pelvis"? You bet I do! While I continually experiment with the latest greatest tools in the nonsurgical POP treatment zone, there is zero doubt I'll be returning to RF. The question is, which other treatment do I partner it with to extend the time frame it lasts? At the end of the day, what women truly want is simply to feel good again, long-term.

> *"All over the world, gynecologists recognize that women do not do Kegel exercises daily as they should. Since I started my practice as a gynecologist in Italy in 1982, the treatment of SUI associated with POP was surgical. Since the 1990s, surgical procedures have changed. Mesh slings replaced Burch, Kelly, and Marshall procedures. Despite good results, the new types of surgery still had potential adverse side effects, such as pain or pain during intercourse. Ten years ago, we started seeing a surge in new nonsurgical procedures that use energy-based devices (EBD). Since I have started treating POP and urinary incontinence using radiofrequency waves (RF) and high-intensity focused electromagnetic wave technology (HIFEM), the results have been outstanding without adverse events. The only downside for patients is they must continue maintenance sessions annually."*
>
> Claudio Catalisano, MD

The one symptom I was hoping would be improved that I have not noticed much change in is intimate sensation. I've read reports of women becoming multi-orgasmic (who doesn't want that, sign me up!), and over the years I've noticed a reduction in sensation which may or may not be related to surgical scar tissue/adhesions or possible nerve damage from childbirth.

I give these treatments a big thumbs up. Based on what I experienced, the improved internal tissue support normalized multiple body functions. My continuing journey has never been about how I look down below; it's about how I feel down below. When we feel healthy, we stand a little taller, walk a little prouder. We clearly need additional research to better understand the value as well as to spark approval by Medicare, enabling the cascade to insurance coverage so women can more readily access this treatment option to improve POP symptoms and restore QOL.

Emsella Chair

BTL's Emsella chair is a high-intensity focused electromagnetic (HIFEM) technology that contracts all the deep muscles of the pelvic floor while you sit in the chair fully clothed. Emsella is said to replicate 10,000 Kegel contractions in a half-hour time frame. Sound like snake oil? This machine is not.

Emsella targets and restores weak pelvic floor muscles to reduce incontinence. When I was first introduced to a magnetic chair for incontinence in 2011, I thought it was a ridiculous concept and reached out to the PT community for opinions, who all agreed it was not worth exploring. However, as pelvic floor treatments evolved, the design improved, and electromagnetic chairs now fill a notable position within the incontinence and pelvic floor strengthening treatment space.

Yes, I have been fortunate to experiment with Emsella chair. Yes, you do remain fully clothed during the treatment. And yes, you will be shocked at how strongly the magnet in this chair contracts pelvic floor muscles. The degree of power (which translates to how tightly your pelvic floor muscles will contract) can be adjusted during treatments, so the intensity is modified to what is appropriate for each individual's needs and tolerance. During my testing mode, I had them increase the energy up multiple times until we hit the top intensity of 10. I was shocked at how strong my contraction became. The treatment was not painful, just felt a bit weird at first because no one contracts the PC muscle that tightly manually. As I moved my buttocks forward and back on the chair, it was abundantly clear to me how the muscles surrounding the urethra or rectum were the primary zones of strongest contraction, priceless considering women with POP navigate both urinary and fecal incontinence.

Add this treatment to your "worth experimenting with" list.

Support Garments

Many women find value in support garments and belts to reduce POP symptoms. The benefit varies depending on type of POP or incontinence, degree of severity, age of user, size of user, and to address the daily ebb and flow of symptoms related to co-existing conditions, lifestyle, and behaviors.

Support garments can be advantageous for women who are experiencing the vaginal or rectal pressure that commonly occurs with POP. POP support garments are typically compression garments made of Spandex, and to be of most benefit for POP symptoms, have 'V' shaped support bands across the abdominal area which push organs and tissues upward. These support garments are much more comfortable and attractive than yesteryear's girdles used to be. They can be washed like other undergarments.

While support garments developed specifically for POP can be purchased online, it is a good idea to initially purchase less expensive support garments locally in a lingerie department to determine whether pressure on the abdomen can be tolerated (some women find the extra pressure against the abdomen uncomfortable). Online versions which be located with a search engine for pelvic organ prolapse + support garments. Some companies now make these garments specifically with POP and incontinence in mind.

Support garments may reduce symptoms in women who are suffering from low back pain, urinary frequency, abdominal strain, or vaginal tissue bulge frustration while waiting for surgery. They also are beneficial for women who prefer to avoid corrective surgery for more advanced POP. Potential benefits are:

- Reduce vaginal pressure and/or rectal pressure.

- Reduce impact of chronic coughing (emphysema, bronchitis, flu).

- Reduce back pain in those who work on their feet.

- Reduce pressure when engaging in general fitness activities.

- Reduce pressure when picking up children.

- Reduce pressure with general daily activities.

- Reduce back pain related to enterocele.

- May reduce stress urinary incontinence, unlikely to help urge urinary incontinence.

- Pregnancy support belts can help both during pregnancy and post-delivery to reduce pressure.

To use a support garment, wash your hands, pull the support garment up to your knees, then lay on a bed or other flat surface. Gently push protruding tissues back inside while lying down, then pull the support garment up until it is in a position at the waist that feels comfortable. The compression provided by the support garment may help contain tissues inside the pelvic cavity until the garment is removed. Obviously, when you pull the support garment down to urinate or defecate, tissues may protrude again from your vagina, so try to avoid bearing down when toileting. Of course, if you are at work, this creates a problem; how do you lay down at work to repeat the entire process? However, many women feel even temporary, short-term support is beneficial.

Vaginal Electrical Stimulation

Your physician or physical therapist may feel that electrical stimulation will be of benefit to improve POP. During clinical electrical stimulation, a small probe is inserted into the vagina or electrodes are placed around the anus and a slight electrical current is applied to the tissues in these areas. A mild electrical impulse generates a contraction that may strengthen muscle fibers. Electrical stimulation may also fire nerves related to urge sensations. Women who have little sensation or muscle strength in their pelvic floor at times can't tell if they are contracting, making it nearly impossible to kegel contract properly or effectively. Electrical stimulation may improve function.

There are also home versions of electrical stimulation available for purchase online without a prescription. Some women may find them beneficial for long-term maintenance post-surgery or possibly to contain POP progression. They may additionally be of value to recharge reduced intimate sensation associated with childbirth or surgical-related nerve damage.

Tibial Nerve Stimulation

The tibial nerve is one of the two branches of the sciatic nerve, the largest nerve in the body. Research indicates an intimate connection between incontinence (both urinary and fecal) and the tibial nerve. Percutaneous tibial nerve stimulation (perforating the skin), also referred to as posterior tibial nerve stimulation (PTNS), is a form of neuromodulation used to treat overactive bladder, urinary urge, urinary frequency, and urge incontinence.

During treatment, a small, slim needle electrode is inserted near your tibial nerve in the inside of the ankle and connected to a battery-powered stimulator. The impulses travel to the tibial nerve and then to the sacral nerve, which controls bladder function.

Treatments occur typically once a week for a 12-week period to monitor improvement of urinary leakage. This treatment is also utilized with a surgically implanted nerve stimulator for fecal incontinence with some success.

Biofeedback

Biofeedback may be used to determine how well your pelvic floor muscles can contract, how well they relax post-contraction, and how long you can sustain a contraction, all beneficial information to have prior to establishing a POP treatment plan. Biofeedback can be used in conjunction with other treatments to monitor improvement of the contractions of the PC muscle. A sensor will measure the contractions of the muscle tissue; it can then be determined if electric stimulation, Kegel exercises, or other treatment modalities are improving the strength of the targeted muscles.

Urethral Bulking Agents

Bulking agents can be injected into the wall of the urethra to reduce the space to assist sphincter closure and decrease stress or mixed urinary incontinence. Although this type of procedure is quick (it only takes a few minutes), until recently the results have typically only lasted 6 months to 2 years and then the treatment had to be repeated.

A newer hydrogel bulking agent called Bulkamid was approved by the FDA in 2020. Bulkamid injections are considered an effective and safe first-line treatment option providing more durable outcomes that have been study-validated to last up to 7 years. This bulking agent may also be of value in patients experiencing occult (post-surgical or sling failure) incontinence or in women with Ehlers-Danlos syndrome weak tissue integrity.

If considering this procedure, request specific details from your clinician regarding what type of bulking agent they utilize, how many of the procedures they have performed, what the success rate is, whether urine retention may occur and if so, for how long, and if there may be an allergic response to the materials used.

Myofascial Release Therapy

The organs and tissues in our bodies are covered in fascia, a thin, tough, elastic type of connective tissue weaving itself around muscles, bones, nerves, arteries, veins, and organs throughout the body, providing structural integrity. Fascia does more than provide internal support; it also has nerves that make it almost as sensitive as skin. Trauma, surgical scars, and inflammation can cause the fascia to tighten, bunch, and stiffen, placing up to 2,000 pounds of pressure per square inch on sensitive structures. Myofascial release massage releases restrictions, improving functionality.

John F. Barnes began teaching the MFR method in the 1970s. His method is characterized by gentle hands-on soft tissue release with prolonged pressure placed on tight, constricted tissue for periods of up to several minutes. Other MFR approaches may use a more aggressive pressure over a shorter time frame; there are multiple styles of soft tissue mobilization. It's valuable for internal and external soft tissues in the pelvic and vaginal spaces to be assessed for restrictions to gently restore proper alignment to the pelvis and coccyx and to decompress any areas of tension around the organs of the pelvis.

To say I was shocked at the difference in my capacity to contract the PC muscle post internal myofascial release therapy (MFR) during my first exploration is an understatement. I was equally shocked during my second MFR exploration at how many internal sore spots existed in my vaginal canal. Much gets lost in translation when describing MFR; you simply have to experience it to better understand the sensations that occur upon release of bunched-up fascial tissue.

MFR can be a valuable tool for treating women's pelvic health issues. Whether exploring MFR as a nonsurgical POP treatment, to maintain post-surgical pelvic health stability, or to level issues related to the complex combination of a hypertonic (tight) pelvic floor and POP, this is a treatment worth exploring.

A qualified MFR practitioner (which may or may not be a women's health physical therapist) should have validated certification. It is a good idea to check with state regulations and screen the backdrop of MFR practitioners prior to exploring the treatment.

7

Surgery

APOPS Patient Perspective: "*Found APOPS and feel so relieved as a 65-year-old needing to mentally prepare for my third surgery in a 23-year span. Great recommendations for pre- and post-op.*"
~DS, California/USA

Nearly everyone is terrified of their first surgical experience. While surgery is rarely a necessity with POP, it is a common patient choice.

Navigating POP symptoms without sufficient relief from nonsurgical treatments can be frustrating. Women who initially hesitate to have surgery and utilize non-surgical treatments often get to the point where POP symptoms become intolerable, particularly the big 4, vaginal tissue bulge, incontinence, chronic constipation, or pain with intercourse. Some women choose to have surgery relatively quickly after diagnosis; they simply can't tolerate the negative impact POP symptoms have on their QOL.

Studies indicate that 13-19% of women will have surgery to repair POP at some point in their lifespan, and approximately 30% of them will undergo a 2nd prolapse procedure. When POP awareness goes mainstream and women recognize symptoms and demand screening, this figure will undoubtedly increase considerably.

The pelvic cavity is an extremely intricate and interconnected grouping of organs, muscles, nerves, and structural tissues. POP surgery improves the anatomical position and function of pelvic organs and most notably, can eliminate or at least radically reduce symptoms. Pain or discomfort can be disabling, but hesitation to go out in public for fear of having an "accident" is a common concern in women who experience urinary or fecal incontinence. Embarrassment about engaging in intimacy with tissues bulging out of the vagina is often the reason women move forward with surgery.

It is important the physician who performs your surgery is a POP subspecialist to ensure the best outcome (gynecologists and urologists are specialists, a urogynecologist is a subspecialist who has received an additional 2-3 years of training in women's pelvic health beyond basic gynecology or urology specialty training).

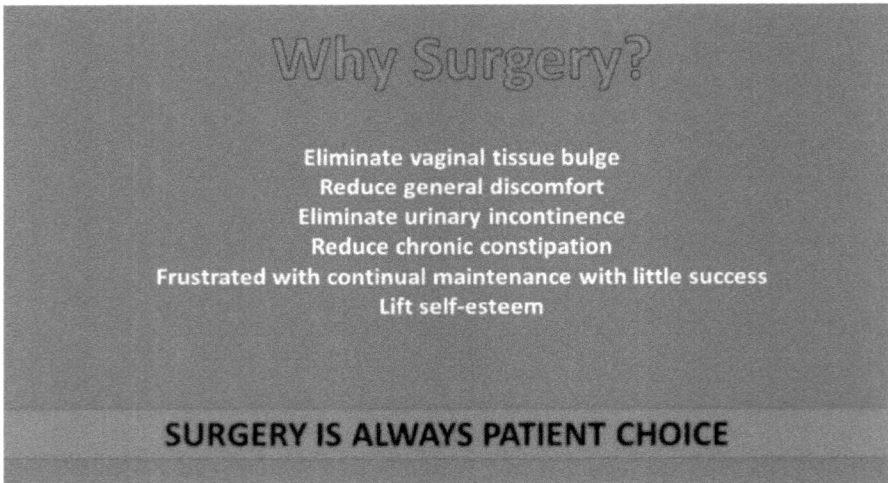

Why Surgery?

Eliminate vaginal tissue bulge
Reduce general discomfort
Eliminate urinary incontinence
Reduce chronic constipation
Frustrated with continual maintenance with little success
Lift self-esteem

SURGERY IS ALWAYS PATIENT CHOICE

Pelvic organ prolapse surgery. Image courtesy of
Association for Pelvic Organ Prolapse Support.

There are multiple types of POP surgeries. Surgical techniques may be transvaginal, abdominal, robotic, or laparoscopic. The type of procedure provided will vary by surgeon. The skillset of the surgeon should be your focal point rather than the technique they utilize. Ask your surgeon how often they utilize the particular type of surgery being recommended. Ask your surgeon to clarify any questions or concerns you have about your procedure.

Mesh may or may not be utilized in your repair. The potential for mesh or other types of complications is greater when appropriate surgical technique is not utilized. POP surgery is optimized when provided by a subspecialist to ensure all types of POP will be repaired with the most appropriate technique possible. A urogynecologist can address all POP issues, providing a one-stop-shop for repairs related to any of the 5 types of POP. This does not mean other types of physicians are not qualified surgeons. It is simply best to utilize the most qualified POP subspecialist to address this extremely complex, variable condition.

Because nearly one-third of POP patients require additional prolapse surgery, polypropylene mesh insertion is a popular consideration to provide long-term surgical success. Native tissue repairs (repairs stitching patient's tissues rather than using mesh) may fail in 1-5 years, requiring repeat surgery. Between 2007 through 2011, transvaginal mesh repair was frequently utilized for POP surgical repairs by surgeons not subspecialty trained in pelvic floor disorders such as POP, resulting in transvaginal mesh complications. Multiple stakeholders gathered in September 2011 for the Food and Drug Administration (FDA) Obstetrics and Gynecology Devices Panel meeting to discuss and determine which surgeons should be permitted to utilize transvaginal mesh, as well as to develop appropriate guidelines. In the interests of achieving the most positive surgical outcome, ask your surgeon to clarify his/her training and experience in utilizing mesh prior to agreeing to surgery that includes mesh. If you have concerns about mesh, the article Mesh Questions to Ask Your Physician is available on the APOPS website or can be referenced in the appendix of this book.

> *"Interestingly, mesh placed behind the vagina through the abdominal or laparoscopic route (the exact same mesh) is still available but is a more invasive and time intensive surgery that was often reserved for women with recurrence, significant apical prolapse, more severe overall prolapse, etc. These procedures have increased overall since vaginal mesh premade kits have been removed from the market. Surgeon training and experience as well as personal results are paramount in this choice. Patients and surgeons must discuss these options specific to each patient's exam, risks factors, and lifestyle, as well as the surgeon's experience, as there is no "one fits all" solution. Unfortunately, many women have been scared by paid television legal advertisements, stories of friends with different surgeries or surgeons, or misinformation about what surgery entails, rather than seeking one or multiple surgical consultations."*
>
> Stephanie Molden, MD

Vaginal mesh provided surgeons and the women they treat a long-term option with higher success over native tissue repairs, and hence why it was brought to market. Unfortunately, the studies mandated by the FDA were stopped prematurely despite no increased harm in those studies and were seemingly based more on public opinion and pressures. Transvaginal mesh is no longer available as a preformed kit or as an option in the U.S.; it requires a discussion between the surgeon and patient regarding the true risks and benefits in other countries.

Activities that occur in the first 12 weeks post-surgery have a significant impact on long-term surgical results. Patients who are extremely active are rarely aware they should modify their behaviors and optimize pelvic floor muscle strength both prior to and post-surgery. It is critical the body has appropriate time to heal post-surgery before attempting to lift heavy weight (including picking up children) or engaging in intense fitness activities. Participating in normal daily activities too quickly after POP surgery increases risk of surgical failure.

The uterus may be removed during POP repair if it is significantly prolapsed and there is no interest in birthing additional children. Uterine-sparing surgical repairs are becoming more commonly utilized for uterine prolapse because undergoing a hysterectomy may increase potential for other types of prolapse to occur.

The removal of the uterus creates an empty space within the abdominal cavity that other organs - particularly the small intestine - can move into. Vaginal vault prolapse (the top of the vagina caves in on itself) is a possibility as well if the apex (top) is not properly anchored during hysterectomy. Like all types of POP, this too can be corrected, but it is important to discuss the possibility of additional prolapses occurring if a hysterectomy is part of the surgical plan. If your gynecologist is providing the hysterectomy rather than a urogynecologist, it is crucial to inquire whether steps will be taken to secure the top of the vagina.

Some women feel a sense of loss when their uterus is removed. Other women are thrilled to no longer need to deal with having a period. Women who hesitate to "give up their uterus" should discuss their concerns with their surgeons or seek counsel prior to deciding whether or not to have a hysterectomy as part of POP repair.

Women are typically informed that POP surgical recovery time is 6-8 weeks. Plan on 12 weeks. While women with less aggressive stages of POP may feel better at 6 weeks, assuming you'll be ready to rock at 6 weeks is a mistake. Often as we heal and become more active, inflammation and what feels or looks like a bulge can reoccur, creating notable pelvic, vaginal, or rectal pressure. Many women fear POP has returned when it is simply body inflammation indicating the need to take activities down a notch.

For all intents and purposes, you want your POP repair to be a one-time fix. Since the incidence of a second surgical procedure for POP is statistically alarming, it is in your best interest to research your surgeon. References are helpful. You can also check physician watchdog websites on-line (check the appendix resources at the back of the book). Check with your state medical board for complaints. However, be mindful that satisfied patients rarely report results online; they simply get on with their lives.

In the past, most POP surgeries were performed under general anesthesia. Currently there is a notable shift in flow, with some urogynecologists providing surgery within their own suites outside of hospitals, utilizing tools and procedures to provide surgery while the patient is awake. Those who have high anxiety about being put to sleep with general anesthesia might want to explore this option if available. There was a time when you would have remained in the hospital a few days after POP surgery, but that is now rarely the case. It is much more likely that you will have a short overnight hospital stay or your procedure will be performed on an outpatient basis, releasing you the same day as surgery. This means you will go home still feeling somewhat rough around the edges. It is imperative you have backup support at home if possible and prep your home prior to surgery with all the post-surgical items you will need.

Recognize that surgical outcome that will depend on the skillset of the individual surgeon, as is the case with any surgery. Most urogynecologists have a preference for specific types of procedures (robotic vs. laparoscopic vs. vaginal vs. abdominal). Your surgeon will discuss your options with you prior to surgery. It is important to do your homework and ask the proper questions regarding types of procedures your surgeon provides, how many they have done, and what the long-term success rate is.

Take as much time locating the best surgeon for your needs as you require; there is seldom a need to rush into POP surgery. Some women seek a second or third opinion in order to find a surgeon that "feels right". Once you select the most suitable surgeon based on your needs, discuss the benefits and risks of each treatment option to enable you to make the most appropriate, informed choice.

8

COLPOCLEISIS: CLOSING THE VAGINA TO OPTIMIZE QUALITY OF LIFE

APOPS Patient Perspective: *"After five different doctors and a pessary that would ultimately fall out, a POP book came to me! Answered all my questions and helped me choose colpocleisis as it had a 90% cure rate. And all the other information in Sherrie's book was so helpful too."*

~BO, Arkansas/USA

If you randomly asked any woman whether she would consider having her vagina sewn shut to eliminate a long-term health issue, she'd likely react with horrified silence. Ask any woman who has suffered for years, and in some cases decades, with the discomfort of vaginal tissue bulge, vaginal pressure, or pain with intimacy that often accompanies pelvic organ prolapse (POP), and you might be surprised at the response. These women simply want to feel normal again, and some are willing to do anything to recapture their former quality of life.

Colpocleisis is a surgical procedure in which the vaginal canal is literally sewn shut to provide internal support to treat bladder, uterine, or vaginal vault prolapse. This highly successful, low-risk procedure is of value for women who no longer have the desire or interest in engaging in vaginal intercourse. It is also upon rare occasions utilized in young women who have additional health conditions that leave them physically compromised and unable to engage in intercourse.

"If you randomly asked any woman if she would consider having her vagina sewn shut to eliminate a long-term health issue, she'd likely react in horrified silence."
~Sherrie Palm

"Pelvic organ prolapse is a complicated condition that has significant impact on the quality and character of a woman's life. The numerous symptoms associated with this condition, which also involve the functions of the urinary, gastrointestinal systems and a woman's sexuality, often present in different ways and are perceived differently based on the life experience of the woman as well as her knowledge of the condition. It is critical that women are given the chance to understand what the contributing factors to this condition are and equally importantly the potential options for care and treatment of this condition with both short and long-term results. Understanding this condition is a key to a successful management and influences the woman's choice for care and caregiver."

Roger Dmochowski, MD

In this procedure, the vaginal opening is literally sealed off with the exception of a small opening to enable secretions to escape. Colpocleisis can be performed using general, regional (spinal or epidural), or local anesthetic. The POP subjective cure rate (based on symptoms) with this procedure is estimated between 90-95%.

Women who are physically fragile and unable to tolerate POP surgery may find this procedure the easiest to recover from. Other women choose colpocleisis because they understand that the vagina is not the core of their sexuality; the brain is. Clearly, intimacy and sexuality can be expressed in multiple ways.

Colpocleisis is a procedure that stands alone in a sea of POP surgical treatment choices. The first report of colpocleisis dates back to 1823 when Gerardin described exposing the anterior (front) and posterior (rear) vaginal walls at the vaginal opening and suturing them together. Geradin's procedure did not include a simultaneous hysterectomy. The most commonly utilized technique is a modification described by Leon Clement Le Fort in 1877, which is a partial colpocleisis with the uterus left intact. Vaginal partitioning is a similar but seldom utilized procedure.

While colpocleisis closes the vagina eliminating the potential for vaginal intercourse, this procedure creates a platform of sorts to shore up fallen organs and tissue inside the pelvic cavity. This eliminates vaginal tissue bulge and pressure. Colpocleisis is most typically utilized to treat POP in women in their late 60s and older. However, in a large database of 4,776 subjects within the Grzybowska 2021 study, colpocleisis was found to have been performed in 47 women between 20–39 years of age to manage advanced POP symptoms that were magnified by other conditions.

This procedure is highly successful long-term and relatively easy and quick to perform in relation to alternate POP surgeries, with the most common risk of complication being a urinary tract infection. No mesh is used in colpocleisis procedures. A very short amount of the vaginal canal is left open, less than 2 inches in length, to enable vaginal secretions to escape naturally. Post-op recovery is relatively quick with minimal discomfort.

The same post-op restrictions apply to colpocleisis as apply to other POP surgeries. While colpocleisis provides a stable internal support platform, women should engage in life-long core and pelvic floor fitness as well as restrict heavy lifting and hard foot strike activities to reduce risk of POP recurrence. It is important to note that colpocleisis is an irreversible procedure. Additionally, if a woman has had long-term non-POP related constipation, colpocleisis is not the fix.

Some women are shocked when they hear this procedure exists. At times women become aware of colpocleisis via "Dr. Google" and dig for more information about the procedure. They can't imagine eliminating a canal that has been a pivotal portal of life and love for the majority of their womanhood. But some women who have suffered extensively from diverse quality of life impacts of POP are relieved they have a non-mesh option that provides a long-term fix.

Women who suffer from Ehlers-Danlos syndrome, a condition that displays as connective-tissue abnormalities and distinctive defects in soft tissue strength, integrity, elasticity, and healing, are predisposed to pelvic organ prolapse and surgical failure as young as their teens. This sector of women may toss the topic on the table with their specialists but are typically denied access because of their young age and little understanding of EDS within general medical practice.

This begs multiple questions. What about a woman's right to choose treatment for her own body? Shouldn't there be consideration of the uniqueness of an adult women's vaginal health needs regardless the age? When women's health issues are the exception rather than the norm, shouldn't healthcare address those needs individually?

A thread querying the needs and curiosities of women in APOPS patient support forum revealed the following questions, which were graciously answered by Vanderbilt University urology subspecializing urogynecologist Roger R. Dmochowski, MD.

· · · · · ● · ● · · ·

Q. IS COLPOCLEISIS OF VALUE TO RELIEVE RECTOCELE OR EN-TEROCELE SYMPTOMS, OR ONLY OF VALUE FOR BLADDER AND UTERUS INDICATIONS?

It helps all elements and can be a real symptom resolver, but women may require simultaneous procedures to address incontinence or posterior repairs, depending on types of POP and grade of severity.

Q. ARE THERE ANY PROTOCOLS TO SCREEN FOR GYNECOLOGIC CANCERS AFTER COLPOCLEISIS?

No, other than an external exam. A pre-operative Pap smear is standard procedure to assure there are no issues prior to surgery.

Q. IF A WOMAN ENGAGES IN HORSEBACK RIDING AND LIFTS HEAVY WEIGHT SUCH AS BAGS OF HORSE FEED, WOULD A COLPOCLEISIS PROCEDURE HOLD UP LONG TERM?

It should. But repetitive heavy lifting is not a good thing after any surgical pro-

cedure, especially regarding the core of the body where a multitude of organs, soft tissues, structural supports, and nerves come together in a very intricate space.

Q. WHAT IS THE APPROPRIATE INCONTINENCE TEST TO HAVE PRIOR TO A COLPOCLEISIS PROCEDURE TO INDICATE AND CLARIFY CONSIDERATION OF A SLING PROCEDURE SIMULTANE-OUSLY WITH COLPOCLEISIS?

Minimally, a full bladder stress test - I personally do urodynamics on all patients given risk of overactive bladder (OAB), and to clarify if the bladder and urethra are performing their job of storing and releasing urine properly.

Q. WOMEN HAVE CONCERNS WITH FUNCTIONAL URINATING AND DEFECATING AFTER COLPOCLEISIS. ARE THERE ANY PO-TENTIAL ISSUES?

If the urinary system is not checked prior to colpocleisis, undetected incontinence may be an issue post-surgery because grades 3 and 4 prolapse may mask this issue.

Q. TISSUE INTEGRITY ISSUES REDUCE POTENTIAL FOR SUCCESS-FUL SURGICAL PROCEDURES AND MAY INCREASE THE RISK OF SURGICAL FAILURE LONG-TERM. IS COLPOCLEISIS AN OPTION A YOUNG WOMAN WITH EHLERS-DANLOS WHO HAS HAD MULTI-PLE FAILED POP SURGERIES SHOULD CONSIDER? AND SHOULD YOUNG POST-MENOPAUSAL WOMEN BE OFFERED THIS OPTION?

It is reasonable to mention but is not generally offered to young women given inability for intercourse post-op. It is always appropriate to offer counseling about long-term irreversible change to female sexuality. Colpocleisis is an alternative POP procedure for the EDS sector to consider for long-term durability, although a fairly radical procedure for young women.

Q. CAN OAB BECOME WORSE AFTER COLPOCLEISIS?

Yes, it can just as can stress incontinence, and patients need to be counseled regarding these issues prior to surgery.

Q. AN ENTEROCELE MAY DROP DOWN INTO THE LOWER PELVIC CAVITY BEHIND OR IN FRONT OF THE UTERUS (OR THE UTERINE SPACE IN WOMEN WHO HAVE HAD THEIR UTERUS REMOVED). WILL AN ENTEROCELE BE ADDRESSED WITH THE COLPOCLEISIS PROCEDURE?

The closure may reduce an enterocele, depending on location. The degree of severity is very individual, so procedures are addressed based on the unique needs of the patient.

Q. IF WOMEN HAVE ALREADY HAD A MESH PROCEDURE, WOULD THAT COMPLICATE A COLPOCLEISIS PROCEDURE?

It could – every woman's situation is unique, so it's difficult to say for sure. It could complicate tissue coaptation (the joining of tissues together in the healing process).

· · · ● · ● · ● · ·

Ultimately as pelvic organ prolapse awareness goes mainstream, women will demand more evolved options. Surgical procedures that show themselves to be effective in the general population will continue. Infrequently provided procedures of value to an appropriate subpopulation such as young women with EDS may be considered more readily. Colpocleisis should be an option more readily discussed and accessible to the women requesting it.

Women are as unique on the inside as they are on the outside, and because lifestyle, behaviors and sociocultural norms vary substantially, it is imperative that we remain open-minded to what individual women need and more importantly, what they want in the way of treatment. But it bears repeating; this procedure will permanently close the vagina. It will no longer be possible to have vaginal intercourse after this surgery. Choice matters.

9

WHEN TO SEEK MEDICAL TREATMENT

APOPS Patient Perspective: *"Pelvic floor health isn't just an "old lady" syndrome to be addressed behind closed doors as a mere afterthought. Education is key. Often times we are too embarrassed to come forward because we think we are on this journey alone. APOPS is breaking through that wall."*

~BV, Indiana/USA

How can we seek medical treatment for a condition that we aren't aware exists? How can practitioners provide appropriate POP screening if they are not sufficiently educated to address it? One of the intentions of this book is to increase awareness of and screening for POP, bringing together patients and practitioners to discuss needs more realistically. Women experiencing symptoms must be encouraged to go to their physicians with questions in hand to spark conversation. Practitioners must be cognizant of and receptive to the very real QOL impact within the POP community.

Early-stage POP does not always cause symptoms pronounced enough or continuous enough to generate concern. The logical way to recognize you may be experiencing POP (or any other medical condition for that matter) is to pay close attention to your body and document the changes you are experiencing to share with your health care provider. But health isn't always logical. Recognize what is normal for you; document changes on a daily basis to understand frequency of occurrence. When you experience a symptom that makes you head to your physician and exams or tests don't clarify the cause, or if symptoms persist or worsen, continue to dig until you find answers.

Since POP isn't a condition routinely screened for, it is possible that your physician may not recognize it or may not be able to determine the type(s) or degree of severity. A POP self-screen may be of value prior to consulting with a practitioner.

It is best to perform this self-test late in the day because POP tends to become most pronounced when pelvic floor muscles become fatigued and gravity has been impacting organ position for multiple hours. To self-screen, go into the bathroom and lock the door to reduce anxiety about being interrupted. Take a hand-held mirror and look for tissues bulging out of the vagina while standing.

If you see tissues bulging from the vagina, share that information with your primary care clinician, gynecologist, or ob/gyn. Once a preliminary diagnosis is made, you will likely be referred to a pelvic organ prolapse subspecialist.

The optimal time to seek treatment for POP is when experiencing symptoms on a repetitive basis or in a pronounced way, such as vaginal tissue bulge, chronic constipation, incontinence, or vaginal and/or rectal pressure. If POP is caught in early stage, nonsurgical treatments can be helpful in reducing symptoms.

> *"Conservative management of POP is related to forces. Ideally, the forces from below the organ are greater than the forces from above, enabling the organs to stay in proper position. If the forces from above are too great (bearing down, poor lifting technique, constipation, weak abdominals and more) or the forces from below aren't strong or stable enough (weak pelvic floor muscles, torn ligaments), organs will shift downward. Women's health physical therapy teaches women to understand how to decrease the forces from above and increase the forces from below."*
>
> Beth Shelly, DPT

If a mild prolapse is diagnosed, it can be monitored while using any of multiple less aggressive nonsurgical treatment options. When POP continues to progress to an advanced stage without diagnosis, there is a strong possibility that surgery may become a significant consideration for repair. Seek additional medical attention when:

- Symptoms become more pronounced.

- New symptoms occur.

- New pain or discomfort arises.

- Unusual vaginal or rectal bleeding or discharge occurs.

It is difficult to judge how often you should see your physician when first diagnosed with mild POP since lifestyle, behaviors, and co-existing conditions that may impact POP severity vary considerably from woman to woman. If prolapse has already progressed to a moderate or severe level, you should consult with a POP subspecialist, particularly if you have pain or discomfort. If the treatments you are using are not effective, your POP may have progressed to the point where you need to consider additional or alternative treatments or surgery.

It is in your best interest to have one surgeon who specializes in all aspects of POP complete all surgical procedures rather than have two different surgeons repairing individual types of POP. Ask your referring physician whom she would use if she needed to have POP surgery. There is often value in seeking a 2nd opinion with an additional specialist. Because POP can impact urinary, bowel, and sexual anatomy, it is of value to check references and do your homework before deciding which surgeon will provide your repair.

10

CHOOSING A HEALTHCARE PROVIDER

APOPS Patient Perspective: *"I found my prolapse at 6 weeks post-partum and started to go down a really dark hole. My OB disregarded this, as this was my new vagina and I had to become my own advocate. I found this group and I wouldn't have been able to survive my first year of motherhood without it."*
~DO, New Jersey/USA

The vagina has been and should be as much a part of women's daily navigation as any other part of our bodies. There is no one-size-fits-all approach to vaginal and intimate healthcare, but there should be a one-size-fits-all objective - enabling women to feel comfortable and confident addressing diverse feminine health needs.

Many distinct types of healthcare practitioners provide treatments of value to women with pelvic organ prolapse from both surgical vs. nonsurgical angles. It is critical to clarify whether practitioners are knowledgeable and certified in women's pelvic floor health concerns. The direction to explore will vary from woman to woman depending on whether nonsurgical treatments to reduce POP symptoms or surgical treatment to fix the prolapse is the objective.

Lack of common knowledge of pelvic organ prolapse makes initial POP treatment navigation confusing. Women rarely know type of practitioner to explore for medical guidance at the onset of their POP treatment journey. Many women think all gynecologists provide the same type of service, simply because that is the only women's health physician they've ever seen. The reality is gynecology and urology provide multiple areas of specialization.

"Pelvic organ prolapse is too simple a name for the constellation of disturbances POP causes the patient. Since it is unpleasant to explain intimacy issues to healthcare providers, women would like to find a single physician to solve all problems in one appointment. However it is our responsibility as pelvic floor surgeons to explain to the patient that often women with POP need guidance from more than one type of well trained, skilled and concerned specialists to manage POP problems. Since a urologist is a "surgeon of the pelvis", particularly the urologist who specializes in female and functional urology, we play an important role in the management of POP symptoms. Furthermore, the participation of the urologist becomes even more essential when urinary tract symptoms are involved."

Carlos Errando-Smet, MD, PhD

Patients are often referred to a Women's Health Physical Therapist to provide insights into pelvic floor anatomy and function and to optimize nonsurgical therapies. Physios have a valuable role to play; they are the soft tissue specialists, experts at educating women about the pelvic floor, how it feels, how it should act, clarifying how lifestyle and behaviors impact pelvic floor health. They often work hand in hand with urogynecologists.

"Physiotherapy has evolved since Arnold Kegel proposed exercises to treat incontinence. The most current treatments include electrical stimulation, manual therapy techniques, postural exercises, breathing exercises, and the use of new technologies such as radiofrequency, biofeedback rehabilitative ultrasound imaging (RUSI), among others. Currently, a physiotherapist trained in the pelvic floor who has all these technologies can design a progressive training program (strengthening, toning loose muscles and relaxing tight muscles) to optimize support of the pelvic floor, while correcting the inappropriate habits that are a risk factor that can make prolapse worse. Additionally, stimulating the production of collagen through radiofrequency is of great value to improve the quality of the soft tissues which, together with the muscles, is crucial when it comes to keeping each vaginal wall and each organ in its optimal position during changes

in pressure that occur during daily living activities, such as coughing or passing stool. For this reason, physiotherapy should be considered essential as a preventive treatment, as a pre-surgery treatment to improve the quality of the tissues when the indication is surgical, and as a post-surgery treatment to prevent recurrence of prolapse."

Inés Ramírez, PhD, PT

Subspecializing gynecologists, urologists, and physical therapists continue their medical training, typically spending 1-3 years focusing on a specific subspecialty field. There are multiple fields of practice within the gynecology and urology sectors:

- General gynecologist (routine care of the female reproductive system, treatment of diseases and disorders specific to women).

- Obstetrician/gynecologists (prenatal care and pregnancy management, diagnosis and treatment of women's reproductive disorders, preventative care, Pap test screening, detection of sexually transmitted diseases).

- Gynecologic oncologists (reproductive-organ cancer).

- Reproductive endocrinologists (hormonal disorders, menopause, pregnancy loss, infertility, and menstrual problems).

- Maternal fetal medicine (high risk pregnancy).

- Female pelvic medicine reconstructive surgeons, both urogynecologists and urologists (functional and anatomical pelvic floor disorders of the muscles, ligaments, nerves, and connective tissues that support the vagina, uterus, bladder, and rectum, particularly pelvic organ prolapse). This is the sector of gynecology most specific to POP.

- General urologist (diagnoses and treats disorders of the urinary tract and stress incontinence).

- Urologic oncology (diagnoses and treats cancers of the urinary tract).

- Neurourology (diagnose and treat bladder dysfunction).

- Female pelvic medicine reconstructive urologist (diagnoses and treats pelvic floor disorders).

- Women's health physical therapists provide baseline screening and treatment for POP; physios with a doctorate in physical therapy have advanced POP training.

Typically, the steps that occur at the primary care or gynecologic level after POP diagnosis are a pessary fitting, referral to a women's health physical therapist for nonsurgical treatment, or a referral to a urogynecologist to evaluate both surgical and nonsurgical options.

A urogynecologist will assess the types of POP you are experiencing as well as the grade of severity and possibly recommend 1 or more tests to clarify how co-existing conditions may complicate your treatment. They may fit a pessary, provide a variety of nonsurgical options, and/or clarify which type(s) of surgery would be the most logical to consider.

A physical therapist can provide insights about and treatment for multiple types of pelvic floor disorders. They assess pelvic floor trauma, muscle tension, coordination, and weakness, and clarify pelvic floor muscle strengthening techniques. They utilize a variety of tools which may include biofeedback, electrical stimulus, ultrasound, heat/cold therapy, myofascial or trigger point release therapy, external and internal soft tissue mobilization, connective tissue manipulation, neuromuscular re-education, bladder/bowel education, postural evaluation, and self-management techniques.

In areas where POP medical providers are scarce, it may be necessary to extend your exploration beyond local providers for treatment options. While a primary care practitioner, general gynecologist, or an Ob/gyn can and do generally provide the initial POP diagnosis, treatment of this condition is very specific and is rarely addressed sufficiently in the general curriculum provided to those fields of medical practice at this point in time. Using the services of a subspecialist whose primary focus is pelvic organ prolapse is a logical direction for POP treatment for those who are not sure whether they want surgical or nonsurgical options since these physicians provide both. Some urologic nurse practitioners, occupational therapists, myofascial release therapists, and biofeedback therapists also specialize in pelvic floor treatments.

You wouldn't trust the care of foot cancer to a podiatrist. It is critical women do their homework and search for a POP subspecialist prior to selecting their healthcare provider. It can provide peace of mind to clarify board certifications. Additionally, it can be priceless to capture patient feedback. Having conversations with women who have walked the walk in a patient support forum can provide considerable information and guidance not available in other formats. Optimize POP treatment navigation from the onset of your journey.

11

POP QUESTIONS TO ASK YOUR PROVIDER PRIOR TO SURGERY

APOPS Patient Perspective: "APOPS *has made me more confident in advocating for myself and teaching my daughter to do the same, because we aren't alone and there is nothing to be embarrassed about having such a common condition!*"

~AR, UK

O nce you make the decision to move forward with surgery to repair POP, a pre-surgical appointment will be scheduled. Prior to this appointment, write down your questions to take along so you don't forget any during the consultation. Your surgeon should answer all questions during your visit. Questions that occur after this visit may be answered by a physician's assistant or nurse practitioner who is typically well-versed in all pre/post-surgical questions. If your surgeon or the PA/NP will not take the time to answer your questions, seriously consider finding a different surgeon. A medical practice that will not readily provide information about the surgical procedure and heal curve is not the best source of quality healthcare.

"Finding a provider to address your pelvic organ prolapse can be challenging! Make sure you feel heard by the provider of your choosing. Seek out a few consultations to make an informed decision for you and your body. Finding a physician who has training in both

sexual health and vaginal reconstruction can be difficult but indeed important."

Michael Reed, MD

Here is a list of suggested questions to consider asking your surgeon. Do not hesitate to ask any question about upcoming surgery; the more knowledge you have going into a POP procedure, the less surprised you will be by events that occur afterward.

1. What types of POP do I have?

2. What is the grade of severity of my prolapse?

3. What type of POP surgical repairs are recommended, rectocele, cystocele, enterocele, uterine, or vaginal vault prolapse repair?

4. Is my prolapse minimal enough that I can maintain it at the same level by doing Kegel exercises and using a pessary?

5. What are the pros and cons of using a pessary as opposed to having surgery?

6. What is the risk of a repeat POP occurrence after I have surgery?

7. What are the surgical risks or potential complications?

8. What type of anesthesia will you use for my procedure?

9. Will I need to stay overnight in the hospital after my procedure?

10. Will the surgery be vaginal, robotic, or abdominal entry? Will there be additional laparoscopic incisions? How many laparoscopic incisions will there be?

11. Will mesh be used for my procedure? Which repairs will mesh be utilized for?

12. What are the risks of erosion if mesh is used to repair my prolapse?

13. How many of the types of procedure you recommend for me have you provided? How often do you provide this procedure? What is the success rate?

14. What are potential complications?

15. How successful is this procedure at maintaining the POP repair long-term?

16. Will this procedure relieve all my symptoms? If not, which symptoms are likely to remain?

17. Will one surgery treat all my POP issues?

18. Will my incontinence be addressed at the same time as my POP surgery?

19. What are other treatment options if I choose to not have surgery?

20. Will I need to wear a pessary after surgery?

21. Will I need to wear an abdominal support belt after surgery if I normally lift heavy objects?

22. How long will I need to be on strong pain medication after surgery?

23. If you find any problems with my ovaries or uterus during surgery, is there a chance that they will be removed?

24. How will this surgery affect my sex life?

25. Will this surgery have an impact on my ability to have an orgasm?

26. How long will it take for sexual sensation to return?

27. Will sex be painful after my surgical repair has healed?

28. How long will I need to wait before I can have intercourse after surgery?

29. How long will it take to get my normal urinary sensations back?

30. How long will it take to get normal defecatory sensations back?

31. How long will I need to wait to return to my normal activities after surgery, including work? What kind of maintenance should I do after I am healed post-surgery?

32. What kind of maintenance should I do after I am healed post-surgery?

Ask all of your questions! There are no bad questions. Any concerns you have should be addressed prior to surgery. It bears repeating; when a physician won't take the time to answer all of your questions or tries to rush you through a pre-surgical appointment, it is a red flag. Search for a surgeon who is willing to address your needs.

12

WHAT TO EXPECT WITH POP SURGERY

APOPS Patient Perspective: *"I knew nothing about POP when I was diagnosed. The APOPS group was my light in what seemed like a very dark tunnel. Thank goodness for all the support, guidance, tips, education, stories, light-hearted moments, and love. It helps so much to know that you are not alone."*

~MS, Australia

Surgery of any type can be frightening and stressful; surgery for a condition that is seldom talked about even more so. Many women with pelvic organ prolapse are so embarrassed to bring vaginal tissue bulge to the attention of their physicians that by the time they do, it has progressed beyond the point of effective management with Kegel exercises or other nonsurgical treatment options.

Clearly, nearly everyone can google for health info. Most women also have friends, family, and work colleagues they can brain-pick about female health concerns. But since women seldom share pelvic organ prolapse experiences, POP information ahead of the curve is rare.

The amount of time surgery will take depends on what repairs need to be addressed, the surgical technique used, and the experience and skill of the surgeon. A routine POP surgery may take between one and two hours; additional time may be necessary for more complex cases. Since some POP procedures address one type of POP and others include multiple repairs, incontinence needs are often a simultaneous surgical procedure. It is best to discuss with your physician the time frame anticipated with your individual surgery.

POP surgeries may include vaginal or abdominal incisions and/or laparoscopic or robotic portals. The heal curve with vaginal, laparoscopic, or robotic procedures will be faster than with abdominal procedures which require cutting through multiple layers of abdominal muscle. Take the time to find a physician you feel comfortable can perform the least invasive procedure for your POP repair. In some cases, there is no choice but to have abdominal surgery. When in doubt, get a second opinion.

After your surgery, it is important to start assisted walking as quickly as the medical staff allows. Sitting up in bed and walking around may be uncomfortable at first. The hardest aspect will be getting into a walking position the first time. Once you are moving around, it gets easier. If you feel too uncomfortable to get out of bed, make the nursing staff aware that you need more medication prior to walking. The quicker you can get up so the blood starts pumping in your body, the sooner the healing process will progress. Your first walk should be prompted and assisted by nursing staff; never try to get out of bed without calling your nurse until you are told it is ok to do so. The last thing you want to do is fall. Injury to a freshly repaired site could be a significant setback.

Women often have a catheter placed after POP surgery; don't be alarmed if this occurs. You may be sent home with the catheter, or alternatively, the catheter will be removed when you are awake and alert, and you will need to urinate after it is taken out before the hospital will allow you to go home without one. If swelling prevents an adequate amount of urine from being released, the catheter will be re-inserted. It is quite common to go home with a catheter for 2-7 days, varying by the complexity of your procedure and degree of swelling. Once internal swelling recedes and tissues start to heal, it will be easier to urinate. You will be instructed about how to use the catheter at home before you are released from the hospital. You will also be told when to make an appointment to come back to your surgeon's office for follow-up needs.

It is a good idea to wear loose-fitting clothing like jogging pants a size too large or bring a loose-fitting beltless robe to the hospital for POP surgery; loose clothing is more comfortable around a swollen surgical site. It will also make the catheter collection bag less noticeable for the trip home. (It will likely be strapped to your leg underneath your pants).

It is relatively common after POP surgery to be sent home with vaginal packing to reduce bleeding and clot formation, although the length of time it is left inside varies by practitioner. Some surgeons do not pack the vagina at all, some leave packing overnight, some leave it in for up to 4 days. The packing is typically removed in your surgeon's office at your first post-op checkup along with the catheter. Instructions on when to make an appointment with your surgeon will be given prior to leaving the hospital.

Catheter and packing removal only takes a few minutes and typically neither procedure is painful, just an odd feeling. At the point both of these procedures are done, you will likely still be on pain medication which will help buffer any discomfort.

Pain is a very individual, personal interpretation. You may be on pain medication for a few days to about a week post-POP surgery; the type and length of time will vary depending on the type of POP surgery you have. It is important to discuss pain concerns with your surgeon *prior* to surgery. Make your physician aware of your level of pain tolerance. If you have any allergic reactions to pain medications, be sure to discuss this with your surgeon prior to your procedure. Icing the surgical sites the first-week post-surgery helps considerably to reduce both pain and swelling. If you feel a sneeze coming on, do not panic; simply grab a pillow, and hold it to your abdominal/vaginal area with gentle pressure while you sneeze. Continual coughing as may occur with a cold may cause discomfort, however. If continual coughing occurs, be sure to contact your surgeon.

Expect considerable bruising and swelling to the entire vaginal area post-surgery. Regardless of the type of incision, this is a major surgery and expect some discomfort. Bruising and swelling may last for a few weeks. Like any other major surgical procedure, the amount of discomfort, swelling, or bruising will vary based on the particulars of your surgical procedure. I was shocked to see a completely black and blue crotch post-surgery, but only because I had not been informed. My colorful black and blue vulval and upper thigh areas were not painful at all.

Around 10 days to 2 weeks following your surgery, the swelling and irritation to the surgical area may increase again. Women often worry the POP "bulge" is back. This swelling is not a cause for alarm; it is occurring because you have returned to your normal daily rituals and are likely moving around more, which causes the swelling to reoccur.

Difficulty urinating and defecating may occur after surgery. Every woman's body reacts a bit uniquely to surgery, especially considering the multiple types of POP surgeries provided. I found that if I urinated a little, then defecated, then tried to urinate again; it gave my bladder time to relax enough to empty completely.

The entire pelvic area will be swollen and sensitive, so do not rush elimination. I felt more comfortable after bowel movements by cleaning the entire region with baby wipes and then lubricating with KY Ultra Liquid after every defecation. A peri-bottle (a bottle to squirt water onto the area) is helpful as well. However, surgical incisions can occur in multiple areas of the perineum. Check with your physician to assure use of any products for cleansing or soothing the perineal area is safe.

It is best to plan on at least 6 weeks off work following POP surgery, although the heal curve can take up to 12 weeks. Since it is relatively common to have multiple POP repairs simultaneously, and since POP repair is in a region of your body that is impacted by standing, sitting, bending over, and walking, it is extremely important that you discuss how much time you will need off from employment when making your surgical plans. The type of employment will determine the length of time before returning to work.

It is likely that your surgeon will ask you to refrain from exercise for six to eight weeks after surgery, and with more complex repairs, it may extend to three months. Heavy lifting and hard foot strike fitness activities should be discontinued until released by your surgeon and realistically should be considered being eliminated from your regimen altogether since they have potential to cause POP recurrence. Follow physician guidelines but pay close attention to body signals when you resume exercising. Pushing into pain post-surgery is never a good idea. At some point, more active women will want to get back to routine exercise regimens, but resuming exercise too soon is truly a mistake. To reduce the risk of a repeat POP repair, you will want to abstain from any form of exercise for the full amount of time your surgeon has designated.

Many women find it takes 8-12 weeks to recover from POP surgery. Those who have the opportunity to take 12 weeks off will find it valuable for healing. Within 3 weeks of surgery, you will start to feel a great deal better but it is important to adhere to your surgeon's instructions. In order to reduce the risk of re-injury, make an effort to avoid pushing, pulling, or lifting motions that put strain on your pelvic floor and cavity.

There are many household cleaning chores that should be eliminated during your heal curve. If you have no one living with you who can help with chores, consider alternate ways to accomplish the things that absolutely have to get handled. Carrying a few items of clothing to put into the washer is acceptable; carrying a laundry basket full of clothes is not. Consider getting a wagon or plastic sled to move items from one end of the house to the other. Your surgeon will give you a weight limit for lifting things around the house, and it is in your best interest to stick to what your surgeon recommends.

There will likely be a bloody vaginal discharge after surgery. It will likely increase in volume after the packing is pulled out. For those women who haven't had a menstrual period in years, it will seem a little unsettling to wear sanitary pads again. After 2 to 3 weeks, you should be able to use a panty liner. If you still need a full pad after this length of time, inform your physician. You should not insert tampons. You truly won't want to; the vaginal area will likely be too tender to even think about using them. You will be able to resume using tampons again, but not until the area is completely healed. This could take three months, possibly more.

You will need to refrain from intercourse for a period of time as well, likely six to twelve weeks depending on your procedure. Most women will not want to engage in sexual activity for at least that length of time anyway; the area will simply be too tender. Recognize the importance of adhering to your surgeon's recommendation on engaging in intercourse; if you become sexually active too soon, it may tear stitches or freshly healed tissue and could undo your repairs.

If the vaginal area seems very dry and irritated to the touch, there are a couple of options to ease the discomfort. Estrogen cream can be very healing to tissues. Women who are menopausal or post-menopausal will likely find applying vaginal estrogen cream to the area helps (estrogen is a prescription item you will need to get from your surgeon). If you normally use vaginal estrogen and use a vaginal applicator to insert the cream, do not use the applicator until the area is healed enough to feel comfortable with its insertion; this will probably be around 6 weeks. Until you are healed enough to use the vaginal applicator, put the cream on the tip of a washed finger and insert it a short distance into the vaginal canal. It may also ease discomfort to apply estrogen cream to the perineum outside the vagina but understand that estrogen impacts your entire body, not just the healing tissues so stick with amounts your surgeon recommends.

Women who are too young to utilize estrogen therapy or who have navigated cancer and must avoid use altogether can apply KY Ultra Liquid to the entrance of the vaginal canal and to the internal areas of the labial folds as well as the rectal area (the liquid works better than the gel for this purpose). Lubricating the entire area after urinating or defecating will help maintain comfort in those first weeks of healing. Do not apply any estrogen or lubricants until your surgeon has released you to do so to avoid contaminating any incision sites. It is also critical when cleaning or applying topical substances to this area to clean or apply from the front of the body towards the back to avoid any fecal contamination to the vaginal area.

If you've had a rectocele repair, you may continue to feel pressure and pain in the anal sphincter area until these tissues are completely healed. Unless there are distinct feelings of great discomfort or pain, the discomfort is likely the normal tissue healing process. During the course of healing, the internal tissues will become a bit hard and rough, but in time, they will soften again.

It is important to maintain soft stools while healing from a rectocele repair. Straining to have a bowel movement impedes the healing process and can damage the repair. Make sure to eat plenty of fresh fruit fiber, especially apples (fruit fiber works better than grain fiber to keep stools soft and consistent unless you are experiencing diarrhea). Use a stool-softener to keep the stool soft enough to evacuate easily; your physician will likely recommend one prior to your release from the hospital. Make sure to take the stool softener every day while on narcotic pain meds. Narcotic pain medication prescribed post-surgery can be extremely binding, and for this reason it is best to get off of them as soon as possible. However, eliminating pain meds too soon is not a good idea. Muscle tissue contracts with pain, which can impede the healing process.

When you feel a bowel movement coming on, lubricate the anus with the KY Jelly (not the Ultra Liquid, in this case KY Jelly will work better). Lubrication will enable the stool to be eliminated more easily, especially beneficial during your first bowel movement. Trust me; you'd rather insert something the size of your finger into your anus to lubricate it than to suffer through a hard, regular-sized stool slowly pushing out. Avoid bearing down to force stool out.

There may be some blood loss from surgery, which may cause iron-deficiency anemia in some women. If you are already taking a supplement with iron, resist the temptation to take an additional iron supplement unless your physician tells you to. Excess iron can cause constipation, compounding post-surgical defecation difficulties. Try to supplement iron from food sources like eggs, red meat, dark green leafy vegetables, or Malt-O-Meal cereal.

> *"We can provide value for every woman with pelvic organ prolapse. While we may not solve all their problems, we can always improve quality of life to some extent."*
>
> Jan-Paul Roovers, MD

Heading into surgery with all your questions answered will reduce fear of the unknown. Share all concerns with your surgeon prior to surgery, and reach out to your surgeon's office with questions post-surgery to optimize surgical outcome.

13

WHAT TO HAVE ON HAND PRIOR TO POP SURGERY

APOPS Patient Perspective: *"I stumbled upon the APOPS group while feeling helpless and alone, searching for information about my condition on the internet. Since then it has been a huge resource of information and emotional support to me. Much love to the APOPS community!"*

~KG, California/USA

I t is of considerable benefit to purchase post-surgical care items prior to your hospital visit so they are readily accessible when you come home from your procedure. Since the length of a hospital stay has shortened considerably over the years and the current dynamic is often day surgery, it is important to have a family member close at hand willing to take care of the needs that would normally be handled by hospital nursing staff.

"All women are entitled to being heard, validated, and supported when making health care decisions. Information and encouragement found through APOPS is a great catalyst for clients seeking answers. Keep asking questions for your own benefit!"

Barb Settles Huge, PT

It is best to have your in-home recuperation area set up prior to your trip to the hospital. Aside from post-surgical items on hand for comfort, there are many additional supplies that will be helpful to make your initial days of healing more user-friendly.

The first thing you will want to set up is your recovery area, whether you will use your bedroom, a spare bedroom, or a couch. Take into consideration the mid-body discomfort you will have after surgery. Your abdominal muscles will likely be a bit unhappy when you first attempt to stand up from your resting position for a bathroom run post-surgery, especially if you have an abdominal incision. Explore which bed location will be the best height for getting into an upright position. Avoid using a recliner initially; there are multiple muscles involved in getting in and out of a reclining chair. Note that the pelvic floor and abdominal area should be allowed to heal before you start intentionally contracting those muscles, so the tissues have time to rebuild properly. Your physician can advise when it is ok to contract abdominal muscles post-surgery, even if you don't have an abdominal incision. Pushing/pulling motions early in the heal curve could be detrimental to the healing process. Your surgeon will likely provide a list of specific restrictions.

An end table or portable TV tray of some kind is useful to put items on that you may need to access in those first day's post-surgery. Make sure your tray area is large enough to keep everything you need within arm's reach. An inverted plastic milk crate available at retail chain stores with an oblong cake pan set on top of a towel to prevent sliding and keep things from falling through the holes works well. An additional hand towel inside to catch the spills may reduce clean-up needs.

There are many other items to consider making your first days at home more comfortable. Give some thought to whether any of the following items may be helpful to you:

- Icepacks are priceless post-surgery to aid pain management and reduce swelling in both abdominal and vulval zones. An acceptable substitute is preemie baby diapers. Open one end and fill with ice cubes and then reseal with the sticky tabs. Since they are absorbent baby diapers, there is no water leakage and the soft inside feels comfortable against the skin. They are very small and fit quite comfortably in the genital curve and on the abdomen. Bags of frozen peas or corn covered with a towel to protect the skin from cold burns work well too, as will a soft cloth-covered beanbag kept in the freezer (can be used for hot or cold). Use icepacks on and off around the clock for the first 4-7 days after you get home from the hospital (ask your physician for guidance regarding time frame, generally 5-10 minutes per hour). I made up two extra icepacks every evening during my first-week post-surgery so when I woke up in the middle of the night needing a fresh one, I simply had to grab it out of the freezer.

- Beanbag-style heating pad is helpful for pain reduction once you get past the first several days post-surgery. It can be heated in the microwave repetitively and there are no electrical cords to navigate. I used a beanbag in both the genital area and across the abdomen similar to ice pack placement. Once I was past the initial four days of icing, I continued with the beanbag heat pad for a few weeks.

- Hydrocortisone 1% cream or hemorrhoid cream for rectal discomfort after your bowels start moving again. Typically, it will be several days after surgery before your bowels become active, and if you've had a rectocele repair, you will want to do everything you can to make the first bowel movements easier. You will not be able to get into a bath to soak for some time, so alternatives to keep rectal discomfort under control are priceless.

- Colace stool softener to ensure the first bowel movement is as easy to pass as possible. Narcotics may be used for pain management after POP surgery, and they cause constipation. Excess iron can cause constipation as well, so if you are using iron for anemia, ask your surgeon whether to adjust your dose. Additionally, surgical blood loss may cause anemia in some women, but rather than using an iron supplement, get iron from natural food sources like spinach, meat, fish, liver, or Malt-o-meal and other enriched cereals unless your surgeon recommends otherwise.

- Apples for fiber will assist the first bowel movement. The soluble and insoluble fiber in apples (with skins on) can be an effective gentle bulking agent and is more effective than grain fiber for constipation, especially for women who struggle with IBS issues or chronic constipation.

- KY Jelly to lubricate the anal canal prior to bowel movements to make evacuation easier.

- KY Ultra Liquid or Liquid Silk will reduce tugging on the external tissues to keep the bottom end more comfortable. Check with your physician about how soon you can use any products near incisions. I found putting KY Ultra Liquid on the entire labial area made me quite a bit more comfortable when I changed sitting or lying positions.

- Foam or inflatable donut will take the pressure off the bottom when sitting for a long time.

- Toddler sippy cup or a child cup with an attached straw comes in handy bedside. It is much less likely to spill if it gets tipped over.

- Cranberry juice is a good liquid to drink after any surgery, as it contains a compound that can inhibit bacteria from attaching to the lining of the urethra or bladder, reducing the risk of a urinary tract infection (UTI). Additionally, drinking a lot of water is essential.

- Sanitary pads and panty-liners are a must. It is normal to bleed vaginally after POP surgery (you may need product for a few weeks, so stock accordingly). If you have vaginal packing, there may be extra bleeding after this is removed, and you will want a pad absorbent enough to handle the flow. After a couple of weeks, you may be able to use panty-liners instead.

- Baby wipes are one of the best innovations ever, handy for so many things. Once bowel movements return, you will want to keep the area very clean to expedite the healing process. Prior to being released by my physician to shower, I found the easiest way to stay comfortable on my bottom end was a series of steps. Initially, clean up using toilet paper. Step two is using a baby wipe to cleanse the area, followed by a small application of hydrocortisone or hemorrhoid cream. I also asked my doctor to prescribe a prescription hemorrhoid cream that had lidocaine in it to numb the area a bit as well as help it heal.

- Loose jogging pants or dresses will likely be the most comfortable clothing; any friction in the vaginal area may create discomfort. I experimented with wearing loose dress slacks and then jeans several times before I was able to tolerate them. Women going back to work at six to eight weeks should experiment at home before wearing pants to work.

- Pain medication will be prescribed by your physician. I recommend that you drop off your prescriptions at a pharmacy on your way home from the hospital. Once you are home and situated, the individual who drove you home from the hospital can pick up your medications. By the time you need your next dose of pain medication, you will have it on hand. It is also a good idea to have whatever over-the-counter anti-inflammatory pain medications you use on hand (check with your surgeon whether to use ibuprofen, naproxen, or acetaminophen). When you are ready to wean off the prescription pain medication, you will have an alternative accessible. I was given naproxen at the hospital along with the narcotic pain medication and continued to use this at home since it stays in your system longer than ibuprofen. Since aspirin may cause bleeding issues, it is best to avoid it to reduce risk of this concern post-surgery.

14

THE MESH MESS: WILL ANXIETY EVER FADE?

APOPS Patient Perspective: *"The holy grail of all things prolapse related! A place where you will learn all the symptoms, all treatment options, and every different outcome possible from real women who have just gone through this life changing event."*

~LI, Arkansas/USA

Y ou've finally taken the steps to approach your Ob/Gyn or primary care physician about your incontinence concerns, the pain you experience during intercourse, and/or the bulge coming out of your vagina. You've been referred to a urogynecologist and have a definitive diagnosis of one or more types of pelvic organ prolapse. Your journey to health balance is now shifting forward. But when the dialogue starts to flow toward whether or not to utilize mesh for repair, you are frozen in fear. What to do?

We all hope our health concerns will be addressed and resolved when having surgical repair. We all hope procedures will be complication-free. Every surgical procedure comes with risk, thus the importance of looking for the best surgeon for your unique surgical needs and the most appropriate type of surgery to optimize results.

It truly takes a specialist to repair the intricate female pelvic cavity, a diverse mass of organs, soft tissues, muscles, ligaments, tendons, boney structures, and nerves pushing against each other in a very compact space. To complicate matters, women with POP typically have more than one type of prolapse in need of repair and each POP type shifts organs from their normal positions. It is kind of like putting an assortment of large, cooked vegetables into a Ziploc bag lying flat on the cupboard. When you hold the bag upright or shake it around, everything squishes together and shifts position.

The controversy regarding the use of polypropylene mesh for surgical treatment of pelvic organ prolapse was quite abundant during the years following the 2011 FDA exploration of mesh complications in the US. Concerns were addressed, system adjustments made, and mesh surgical treatments moved forward. However, regulations surrounding the use of mesh implants vary by country. Unfortunately, the world at large did not follow suit with US action in 2011. Transvaginal mesh complications (vaginal insertion of mesh) continued to occur overseas, particularly within the UK through 2019.

The use of transvaginal mesh implants for POP and urinary incontinence was extensively debated among experts as well as the general public in 2019. USA, UK, Canada, Australia, New Zealand, and France have removed transvaginal mesh implants for POP from the market. They remain a surgical option in most mainland European countries, Asia, and South America. Rely on your POP-specializing surgeon to advise which surgical options are accessible to you.

> *"Unfortunately, there were not enough data at the 3-year fixed FDA timeline in 2019 to prevent the decision to remove transvaginal mesh kits for POP from the market in the U.S. We have now learned in subsequent studies that followed patients for 5 years that transvaginal mesh products can be superior to native tissue repairs. It is a shame that patients do not have those options available to them anymore in the U.S."*
>
> Charles Nager, MD

While much has been addressed to improve the outcomes of mesh procedures, fear factor remains high for many women who remember the barrage of litigation commercials shown on television. Mesh complication media exposure during both 2011 and 2019 time frames rarely provided balanced information on both the pros and cons of mesh. Media focused on the negative spin of complications, generating significant fear factors for women heading into POP surgery. Seldom do women who've had successful mesh procedures (the majority of procedures) talk about them; they simply get on with their lives. Let's revisit the purpose and value of mesh treatment for pelvic organ prolapse, as well as share insights on best practice techniques utilized by urogynecologists.

Every woman navigating POP would like to have a magic list of "the best of the best" when it comes to pelvic floor clinicians. Unfortunately, it is not that simple because needs differ significantly from woman to woman. Surgeon skill set, mindset, and personality are as individual as the patients they treat; practitioners are human after all. Some women prefer the most skilled surgeon, with little concern about bedside manner. Some women prefer great bedside manners but may be disappointed that the surgical outcome is not perfect or the healing took longer than expected. Ideally, women can locate a highly skilled surgeon with both exceptional skill and great bedside manner. The skill set of clinicians will obviously vary with time, experience, and continuing education, as well as adoption of new innovations and tooling.

If considering mesh surgery, it is important to find a surgeon with extensive mesh experience. Write down the questions you want to ask your doctor before your appointment to make sure you don't forget any. Let your practitioner know you have anxiety about mesh surgery if that is the case. Ask your surgeon what steps they take to avoid mesh complications. Small incisions, proper mesh insertion location, preparation of mesh insertion site, use of estrogen cream pre- and post-surgery, degree of mesh tension, and an appropriate closure are important considerations for a quality mesh procedure, whether your surgeon performs mesh surgery through a transvaginal, laparoscopic, robotic, or abdominal approach.

It is a red flag when clinicians or industry magnify the benefits only of a product or procedure. You should hear both sides of the story, risks and benefits, in order to be fully informed and better enabled to make the most appropriate decision regarding whether to move forward with surgery. My POP procedure in February 2008 was transvaginal, and a consultation with my urogynecologist in 2015 at 7 years past that surgery confirmed that my tissues remained healthy, the mesh was in proper position, and there was no erosion. At the time of publishing this book, I have reached the 15-year post-mesh procedure point with no mesh or surgical complications that I am aware of. I am grateful mesh was an option for my surgery, and finding the right subspecialist is priceless. Obviously, there is never a 100% guarantee of success with any surgery, but if all of your questions are answered, it will give you peace of mind heading into a procedure.

It is important to understand that mesh is typically used to prevent additional POP surgery down the road. Without mesh, surgery may fail in one to five years if our own tissues are not strong enough to maintain the repair long-term. It should not be surprising that lifestyle, behaviors, co-existing conditions, and the aging process increase risk for repeat surgery, especially given how active the average woman is. While childbirth is absolutely the most common POP cause, most women have a multitude of additional risk factors. Show me a woman with one cause alone and I'll show you a woman who is the exception to the rule.

The diagnosis and management of pelvic organ prolapse will evolve considerably over the coming years. While APOPS pushes behind the curtain to engender broad-spectrum awareness and elicit POP screening standardization in pelvic exams, research continues to brainstorm causal links and risk factors, and practitioners evolve skills regarding advanced treatment options. Patients, practitioners, and researchers continuously learn side by side.

Locate urogynecologists in your area and google them individually to see what information you can capture regarding procedure experience, length of time in practice, and what services they provide. Physician review websites will give you basic information to start with but are not a 100% guarantee of practitioner quality. It is imperative to dig deeper and possibly consider meeting practitioners in person to decide whether your unique needs will be met. Pelvic organ prolapse is a condition that absolutely warrants a second opinion if you are not comfortable with the first subspecialist you see. While surgical skill is a top priority, a practitioner who answers your questions and understands your specific needs is priceless.

A well-informed patient will have less anxiety and greater opportunity for the best outcome. As patients, it is our responsibility to do our homework. Check references, get referrals, and consider second opinions. POP treatment is diverse, complex, and continually evolving. It is critical women ask all of their questions about surgery in general and about mesh specifically and not move forward with surgery until receiving all answers needed to understand surgical options. A list of mesh questions to consider asking your surgeon prior to POP surgery is accessible by referring to the appendix of this book or googling APOPS + *Mesh Questions to Ask Your Physician.*

APOPS mesh stance has been and at this point in time continues to be women should have the right to choose whether or not to utilize mesh. Following are the speeches provided at the FDA mesh meetings in 2011 and 2019 in representation of APOPS' stance on patient pro-mesh choice.

2011 Mesh Presentation To The FDA Panel

The following speech was given in Washington, DC by Sherrie Palm to the FDA OB/Gyn Advisory Panel Addressing Transvaginal Mesh Protocol on September 8, 2011, in representation of APOPS' position on the value of transvaginal mesh procedures for repair of pelvic organ prolapse.

"I'm Sherrie Palm, the founder and president of the Association for Pelvic Organ Prolapse Support. Neither me nor APOPS has any financial relationship with any person or group involved in any POP mesh agenda. I am simply a woman who's had transvaginal mesh surgery to repair pelvic organ prolapse. I had 3 of the 5 types of POP. I am a success story and would like to share some insights with the committee members. Like most women, I'd never heard of POP prior to my diagnosis. My urogynecologist utilized a transvaginal mesh procedure for my surgical repair. I had concerns about repeat surgery if mesh was not utilized, an all-too-common occurrence. I've been extremely pleased with the outcome of my surgery for pelvic organ prolapse and I guide others daily how to investigate the benefits of locating a specialist in POP procedures.

As a women's pelvic floor health advocate, I truly felt the need to weigh in on this topic. It's vital that committee members recognize that the common denominator for all women is the desire to return their bodies to normal. This is what drives women to seek treatment including surgery for POP. All women with POP have symptoms. ALL WOMEN WITH POP HAVE SYMPTOMS; they just don't talk about them with their physicians, husbands, even their friends; they are simply too embarrassed - but they talk to me. I speak with women daily regarding the baggage that comes with pelvic organ prolapse.

I'll admit that I'm a bit more proactive than the average woman. I networked to find the best urogynecologist in my area. I checked her credentials. I went to my appointment with my questions in hand with no intention of leaving until all of my concerns were addressed. My physician is an expert in her field. She took her time with me, and my successful transvaginal mesh procedure substantiates that this treatment option does have great merit.

I recognize that few women do their homework when approaching POP treatment; because of that some women have transvaginal mesh procedures performed by physicians without the proper training and expertise for this procedure. With so many organs, muscles, and connective tissues coming together in a tightly compacted area, it truly takes an expert to get it right. A female pelvic medicine urogynecologist or urologist should be the physician of choice.

When the efficacy of a medical procedure is questioned, the catalyst typically comes from complaints filed by individuals who suffer complications after having procedures by physicians with inadequate training or experience. My heart goes out to the women suffering from mesh complications; it truly does. I've spent time discussing their histories with them and it is vital that we listen to their voices. These are women who had pain and dysfunction, opted for surgery to correct the issues, and now their pain and dysfunction are compounded. However, eliminating this beneficial procedure from POP treatment options is not the answer. Monitoring who can perform procedures is a more practical direction. Advancement of any medical pathway will always be littered with the "yikes" factor of those who add procedures to their itinerary as though picking up a tool at Home Depot. It has always been this way; it probably always will. Thankfully we have the FDA to monitor and create ballast.

I feel strongly that transvaginal mesh procedures should be recognized as a valuable option in the choices for pelvic organ prolapse treatment. I also feel strongly that these procedures should only be utilized by physicians who are specialists and have gone through the intensive training necessary to perform them. I am hopeful the FDA will consider monitoring the training protocol rather than preventing urogynecologists from performing transvaginal mesh procedures. It's likely that the majority of the complications that occur are the result of inadequate training and experience. POP surgery is best left to the experts.

As a women's pelvic floor health advocate, every aspect of impact POP has on women is of top priority to me, every single layer. Transvaginal mesh is just one of them. Pelvic organ prolapse is not an American women's health issue; it is a global women's health pandemic. There are 3 million women in this country alone with POP. It is imperative that the FDA is intricately involved in the global path to proper diagnostics and treatment for POP, along with coordination from NIH and WHO. Forward thinking will address the perception of POP as well as the reality of the status quo in all matters POP related including transvaginal mesh."

2019 Mesh Presentation To The FDA Panel

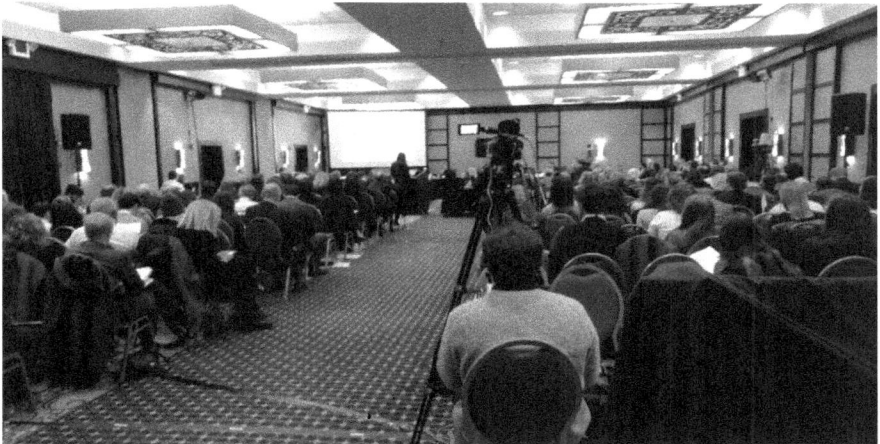

FDA Ob-Gyn Devices Panel Meeting, 2019. Image courtesy of Association for Pelvic Organ Prolapse Support.

Following is the speech given by Sherrie Palm at the FDA Obstetrics and Gynecology Devices Panel Transvaginal Mesh Meeting on February 12, 2019.

"I'm Sherrie Palm, the founder of the Association for Pelvic Organ Prolapse Support (APOPS). Neither me nor APOPS has any financial conflicts of interest. In full disclosure, I am a transvaginal mesh success story, 11 years post transvaginal mesh cystocele and rectocele repair and native tissue enterocele repair.

Pelvic organ prolapse is not an American women's health issue; it is a global women's health pandemic. Since 2010, APOPS has been engaging with women, healthcare, academia, research, industry and policy, a 177-nation strong network. The women we serve are mid-teens through end-of-life, navigating every diverse POP issue, including the mesh vs. native tissue debate. APOPS has considerable following in the UK and Australia; obviously mesh comes up regularly.

I submitted documents to the committee, but I also wanted to give voice to the voiceless today - the women who have had successful transvaginal mesh surgery. The majority of the women in our space who have mesh are happy with their procedures and move on with their lives rather than engage in the hostile energy quite prevalent in anti-mesh forums and the media.

Everyone attending this meeting is aware that POP has pandemic-like prevalence of 40-50%. The stigma of pelvic organ prolapse symptoms continues to shroud POP in silence despite nearly 4,000 years on medical record. I implore the committee to analyze mesh controversy through a progressive lens. Millions of women experience POP; millions will need surgery in coming years. I assure you that behind APOPS curtain, women are becoming empowered and vocal. And they deserve treatment options.

Consider the ramifications of POP awareness going mainstream as the result of media exposure clarifying POP prevalence, symptoms, and quality of life impact on a program such as 20/20.

Consider the ramifications to healthcare, the insurance industry, policy, and women's wellness protocol that will arise if 30% of the millions of women having surgery need repeat procedures because mesh is no longer an option.

And consider the ramifications of women needing repeat surgery but who choose to forgo it because they don't want to replicate the discomfort, expense, and downtime of prior failed procedures (note plural, often women need more than one repeat procedure post native tissue repair).

The evolution of healthcare typically follows a long and winding road, often under construction.

Unfortunately, in medicine, we don't know what we don't know, and the nature of healthcare, as in any other system, is to evolve step by step. It is imperative throughout this process that patient voice continues to be enabled and respected to effectively and efficiently identify issues that must be addressed, and that includes the voices on both sides of the mesh debate.

As I mentioned at the FDA meeting in 2011, my heart goes out to the women with mesh complications. I've spent considerable time communicating with many of them, and it is pivotal that we listen to their voices. However, eliminating beneficial procedures from POP treatment options of value to the majority of women is not the answer.

We must not let overseas energy influence due process stateside. The health status of millions of women hangs in the balance of decisions made by this committee. I implore the committee to consider the voices of the silent majority and to recognize that as a country, we have and should continue to move forward, addressing issues, leading the global charge to evolve best practices. There is no doubt the next significant evolution of women's pelvic health screening, treatment, and wellness directives looms large. It is APOPS' opinion, as well as my humble opinion, that transvaginal mesh, including for cystocele repair, should continue to be an option on the table. Every Voice Matters."

OUT OF SIGHT QUALITY OF LIFE IMPACTS

15

THE IMPACT OF ATROPHY: WHEN PAIN REPLACES THAT LOVING FEELING

APOPS Patient Perspective: *"I'm so glad there's finally forward momentum toward open, comfortable discussion of women's vaginal health. APOPS is leading the global drive."*

~LB, Utah/USA

W ho doesn't want a physically and emotionally fulfilling sex life? POP symptoms such as tissues bulging out of the vagina and pain with intimacy are far too often roadblocks to sexual bliss. While the emotional distress women experience when tissues and organs misbehave during sex-play may hinder engagement, pain with intimacy can shut the door completely.

As common as vaginal atrophy is, it often persists untreated, creating a desert in a formerly moist environment. The sandpaper effect during intercourse falls far short of pleasurable. Intimacy often stops altogether because women can't tolerate the pain. Effective communications between intimate partners can't occur regarding atrophy when women aren't familiar with what atrophy is or why it occurs.

Estrogen loss related to menopause and perimenopause is considered the 2nd leading cause of POP. Beyond the loss of muscle tissue strength and integrity, estrogen depletion as we age may result in vaginal and vulval tissue atrophy, causing tissues to become irritated, thin, dry, and less supple. Vaginal secretions are reduced, resulting in decreased lubrication during sex. Dry, itchy, fragile vulvovaginal tissues are susceptible to injury, tearing, and bleeding during intercourse. Intimacy may become so excruciating that sex is avoided altogether. When a woman does not engage in intercourse regularly during and following menopause, the vagina may become shorter and/or narrower, causing pain when intercourse is attempted, even when using a lubricant. Atrophy can be a considerable roadblock for women already struggling with POP-related self-esteem issues. The impact on sexual satisfaction and relationships can be devastating.

"Women experience the most dramatic impact of estrogen deficiency with menopause, mostly with serious complaints of the urogenital system. 'I feel like my vagina is on fire, it is an unbearable pain', 'having sexual intercourse is now a nightmare', 'I get cystitis very often', 'I am tired of taking antibiotics', 'my vagina hurts even while sitting', are the most common complaints I usually hear from my patients. They usually try to solve these quality-of-life complaints either by using their own home-grown method or trying to deal with vaginitis and/or cystitis treatments that are often prescribed to them.

I try to explain the importance of vaginal estrogen cream use by telling them just as we constantly protect our hands or face and lips from dryness, cracking, and aging by using various creams; the vagina should be moisturized and strengthened with the same care to decrease the impact of atrophy. Even the application of estrogen-containing creams to the vagina once a week from the very beginning of atrophy can protect the health, flexibility, and tone of the vagina and prevent many problems that may occur.

The most important role for the physicians is to emphasize the importance of using local estrogen creams in the management of menopausal genitourinary syndrome and to explain to their patients that its use will not only improve sexuality for menopausal women who have poor or no sex life but that it is essential as it protects the health of the vagina and lower urinary system, without any adverse effect."

Fulya Dökmeci, MD

When POP and atrophy tag team, it magnifies symptoms and complicates care. A woman with POP who is experiencing pain may attribute the pain to POP when in actuality, it is the dry irritated vaginal tissues causing the pain. Estrogen is priceless to the POP heal curve both pre- and post-surgery, plumping up and moisturizing tissues, aiding the recovery process. When a woman is a few weeks post POP surgery and is still experiencing notable pain, it is of value to check hormone levels to clarify if atrophy is the pain source rather than the surgical repair.

Atrophy can be a roadblock, whether we are evaluating it from the physical, emotional, sexual, or surgical angle. Aging does not mean you have to put up with atrophy. Treatment for cancer does not mean you have to put up with atrophy. Lack of sex drive does not mean you have to put up with atrophy. And certainly, when a POP surgery has "gone well" and pain continues, estrogen may be your best friend.

16

WHAT IS VAGINAL LAXITY? THE CULTURE OF SILENCE IN VAGINAL HEALTH

APOPS Patient Perspective: *"After being diagnosis with POP at 34, I was so distraught. APOPS helped me to understand that I am a part of a huge movement, and I feel so much more empowered in both my personal journey and my health career."*

~LR, North Carolina/USA

V aginal health is of notable significance in terms of women's sense of sexual wellness but is rarely an openly acknowledged or discussed aspect of women's health. Females typically put their health needs last, whether they are CEOs of large corporate entities, clerks at Walmart, stay-at-home moms, or deeply embedded in medical practice.

Vaginal laxity is an overlooked, often cryptic aspect of health many women find bothersome. Why can't women bring themselves to talk out loud about vaginal laxity or the "gap", the wide vaginal opening and stretched-out internal tube of vaginal space that typically occurs after vaginal birth? Vaginal laxity impacts sexual sensation, and women not only have less satisfying sexual experiences, but they also worry whether their partners are satisfied. Women ponder whether their vaginal opening is unattractive and may be a turn-off for their intimate partners. The gap impacts women's self-esteem in ways that seldom make it into sexual conversation with intimate partners. Gap conversations rarely occur during pelvic exams.

Both patient and practitioner input is imperative to provide balance to this most pivotal conversation about women's wellness and sexuality. To lift the shroud of secrecy, let's dive a bit deeper into this aspect of vaginal health. Kicking off the conversation is an empowered woman in her 30s. Melissa explored options to treat pelvic organ prolapse and simultaneously address vaginal laxity and gap concerns. Adding balance to the discussion is cosmetic gynecologist Marco Pelosi III MD.

· · · · ●·● · · · ·

Q. MELISSA, PLEASE SHARE YOUR POP HISTORY, AGE OF PELVIC ORGAN PROLAPSE ONSET, AGE OF DIAGNOSIS, THE CAUSE OF YOUR POP.

I suspect I had a very mild rectocele after giving birth vaginally the 1st time at 29. Never diagnosed, but I did sometimes need to splint to have a bowel movement. I was diagnosed with retroverted uterus when I was pregnant with my 2nd child at the age of 31. After giving birth vaginally the 2nd time at the age of 32, I was diagnosed with rectocele. Childbirth was the cause, although I used to do some heavy lifting as a Pre-K child educator, which I had to give up once I was diagnosed.

Q. DID YOU SELF-DIAGNOSE, OR WAS YOUR POP DIAGNOSED BY YOUR OB/GYN?

I was diagnosed by my ob/gyn when I went in 10 days post-partum due to severe constipation.

Q. WHAT TYPE(S) OF POP DID YOU HAVE?

I was diagnosed with rectocele. I later found out there was an enterocele too, and slight bladder and uterus prolapse as well.

Q. WERE YOU FAMILIAR WITH PELVIC ORGAN PROLAPSE PRIOR TO YOUR DIAGNOSIS?

I researched POP when I was first having to splint to have a bowel movement after giving birth to my first child. I had never heard of it before that.

Q. WHAT TREATMENTS HAD YOU TRIED TO TREAT YOUR POP?

I tried physical therapy and found it unhelpful and painful. I then had surgery at 3 months postpartum for the rectocele. When they went in, they wound up having to fix the enterocele instead. I read this in my notes a year later, was never told they changed the procedure. I saw no improvement in symptoms (constipation, urine leakage, painful sex).

I tried an OTC pelvic muscle exercise device but found it only helped with urine leakage, not prolapse.

I tried a pessary, but it was painful (caused severe rectal pressure) and I was unable to have a bowel movement at all with the pessary in. It pinched off the path.

Then I used a sea sponge as a pessary. It was more comfortable, but it got stuck in position and I had to have it removed by a gynecologist, who told me it was not a good idea to put sponges in your vagina. She suggested a mesh bladder sling, which I did not want.

I tried multiple pharmaceutical medications for incontinence and constipation.

I tried vaginal estrogen.

I finally had my 2nd surgery 18 months postpartum.

Q. WHAT REPAIRS WERE INCLUDED IN YOUR SURGERY?

My first surgery at 32 included native tissue enterocele repair (instead of the planned rectocele repair). My second surgery at 34 included an abdominal laparoscopic non-mesh bladder lift, hysteropexy uterine suspension, vaginal rectocele repair, perineum repair, labiaplasty (labia was partially torn off during childbirth and needed to be reattached), and vaginoplasty.

Q. DID YOU CONSULT A UROGYNECOLOGIST, AND IF SO, AT WHAT POINT?

I saw a urogynecologist who was also a cosmetic gynecologist at 18 months postpartum. I traveled 5 hours to Atlanta to see him. I sought treatment from a local aesthetics surgeon first who only offered laser vaginal rejuvenation and to his credit, admitted it does not provide a permanent fix for prolapse. He also told me he could only remove my labia, not re-attach it.

Q. WAS INTENT OF VAGINOPLASTY TO REPAIR POP OR TO ADDRESS THE GAP AND IMPROVE YOUR SENSATION & INTIMATE RELATIONS?

The vaginoplasty portion of the procedure was to improve sexual function. The other procedures I had along with it addressed the prolapses. The bladder lift, hysteropexy, and other repairs were covered by insurance. The labia re-attachment and vaginoplasty were not.

Q. HOW DID THE PROCESS OF CONSULT GO FOR VAGINOPLASTY?

When I arrived at check-in, they gave me a small slip of paper and asked me to please answer this question: "Are you interested in a vaginal tightening procedure?" I checked yes. I saw the doctor; he stated I had multiple prolapses, and he was surprised I'd already had a repair; he said it didn't look like they'd fixed anything. I got dressed and met him in his consult room with my husband. He described all the procedures to fix the prolapses, and I said okay to all of those. He then sent in a female office employee to discuss the vaginoplasty; she basically said it would be $6000 out of pocket and gave us a credit application. My application was approved, and they added vaginoplasty to the procedures. I asked about labiaplasty at this time, and that was also added to my list of procedures.

Q. HOW LONG WAS YOUR HEAL CURVE WITH THE MULTIPLE PROCEDURES?

It took me 14 weeks to heal enough to go to work. It took 8 months to heal enough to have intercourse.

Q. HOW PAINFUL WAS THE HEAL CURVE?

It was virtually painless because I was fortunate enough to be able to take time off work and just lay down a lot. I was also on opioid pain medication for 3 weeks.

Q. DID YOU ALLOW YOUR HUSBAND TO VOICE AN OPINION ABOUT WHETHER YOU SHOULD HAVE PROCEDURE OR NOT, OR WAS IT YOUR DECISION SOLELY?

My husband realized I wanted the procedure badly, and he supported it for that reason. He never pressured me to have it. It cost a lot of money, and I was hesitant to spend that much, but he was vocally in favor of the repairs, so I felt okay about doing it. Sex was too painful for me in the two years between my 2nd birth and my procedure, so we weren't having any at all. We really had nothing to lose and everything to gain.

Q. ARE THERE ANY QUESTIONS YOU WISH YOU HAD ASKED YOUR SURGEON?

I don't really have any questions I wish I'd asked because he was so prepared and told me everything I needed to know before my repairs. I do wish I'd asked my first doctor more questions, as maybe if I'd known he couldn't do anything to fix a rectocele or restore sexual function I would have skipped that operation and only had surgery once.

· · · · ● · ● · ● · · ·

INSIGHTS FROM MARCO PELOSI III MD:

Q. WHEN A WOMAN CONSULTS WITH A COSMETIC GYNECOL-OGIST WITH COMPLAINTS OF LACK OF SEXUAL SENSATION BE-CAUSE HER VAGINA IS TOO LOOSE, DOES THE PHYSICIAN ASSESS INTROITUS, VAGINAL CANAL, OR BOTH?

A properly trained cosmetic gynecologist would check all of these areas. However, in my world, a qualified cosmetic gynecologist is also really good at urogynecology. The never-ending problem though is that there are many pretenders who call themselves cosmetic gynecologists and know zero about urogynecology and vice versa.

Q. DOES THE SIZE OF THE "GAP" AT THE INTROITUS INDICATE THE WIDTH OF THE ENTIRE VAGINAL CANAL OR JUST THE ENTRANCE SIZE?

The vagina is shaped like a funnel. The introitus is the mouth of the funnel. I measure the dimensions at the introitus and at the mid-vagina levator region separately. They represent different muscle groups.

Q. CAN VAGINAL LAXITY OR WIDE VAGINAL GAP AT THE INTROITUS CONTRIBUTE TO LESS SUPPORT OF PELVIC ORGANS, THUS IMPACTING PELVIC ORGAN PROLAPSE DEGREE OF SEVERITY?

Absolutely. The question you are asking is "What is the function of the perineum?" The perineum is that last structure between the pelvic organs and the outside world. And if that structure is broken, your pelvic organs are headed on an unplanned trip to the outside world.

Q. PLEASE DESCRIBE HOW COSMETIC REPAIRS TO ADDRESS VAGINAL LAXITY OR WIDE INTROITUS DIFFER FROM A TRADITIONAL A&P (ANTERIOR/POSTERIOR PROLAPSE) REPAIR.

Cosmetic repairs are focused on reducing caliber at the level of the muscles. Traditional repairs are focused on lifting vaginal supports at the level of the fascia. They don't address muscles or caliber in any meaningful way.

Q. IF A WOMAN HAS LEVATOR DAMAGE FROM CHILDBIRTH, AND HAS VAGINAL LAXITY AS WELL, WOULD ADDRESSING LAXITY PROVIDE SUPPORT TO THE ORGANS?

What you are asking in essence is does a levatorplasty provide pelvic floor support? It does do a degree, but not enough. This would be tantamount to skipping a rectocele repair and substituting a muscle repair instead. This was tried for over a half-century with aggressive muscle repairs and the result was severe pain and high failure rates. For more information to clarify, Google ISCG + they are wrong about levatorplasty.

Q. DO YOU FEEL VAGINAL LAXITY WILL EVER BE CONSIDERED AN ESSENTIAL INSURANCE-COVERED PROCEDURE (VAGINAL HYPERLAXITY SYNDROME?) IF THIS REPAIR PROVIDES SUPPORT FOR THE PELVIC ORGANS?

When lousy sex is considered a medical problem and when surgery for lousy sex is considered a medically indicated treatment for its management (pigs will be flying at this point), then perhaps medical insurance companies might cover this. However, since the correction of vaginal laxity doesn't support the pelvic organs, that would never be a basis for getting it covered.

· · · ● · ● ● · · ·

Why are vaginal and intimate health shrouded in silence? Why does the world at large continue to find it awkward to talk about these pivotal aspects of women's health out loud? When we overcome this last significant barrier to female empowerment, women's health will finally be set free.

17

EHLERS-DANLOS SYNDROME: A CO-EXISTING CONDITION THAT COMPLICATES CARE

APOPS Patient Perspective: *"Don't treat me like I'm some kind of web-browsing-self-diagnosing-wackadoo-hypochondriac. I know my own body; I've had it my whole life!"*

~LL, PA/USA

Within the POP patient community, there is a co-existing condition that complicates care considerably more than others, Ehlers-Danlos syndrome. EDS is one of the most frustrating and least recognized intersects a select group of women with POP experience. EDS displays as joint hypermobility (more commonly called "double-jointed"). More significantly, it presents as exceptionally stretchy or fragile skin that bruises and tears easily externally and provides little structural integrity internally.

EDS is a group of multisystem disorders that affect connective tissue throughout the body in diverse ways. There are 13 subtypes of EDS that include a variety of symptoms and severity. Most of the EDS categories are rare. Considered the most common systemic inheritable disorder of connective tissue, hypermobile EDS (hEDS) and the related Hypermobility Spectrum Disorders (HSD) are estimated to represent 80-90% of EDS cases. The EDS subtype hEDS is the most typical POP/EDS overlap.

Despite noteworthy occurrences, the intersect of EDS and POP is rarely recognized during routine women's wellness exams. There is a considerable need
to broaden an understanding of weak tissue integrity and how that accelerates
POP manifestation and development. Given the fact that EDS curriculum is not
a standard aspect of gynecologic study, it's no shock that the women's wellness
medical community does not recognize it.

While accurate prevalence data currently doesn't exist for EDS or POP, research
estimates EDS occurs in 1 in 5000 people with approximately 70% prevalence in
females. POP is a noted condition included within various EDS classifications.

> *"When I think about causes of pelvic organ prolapse in young pa-
> tients, the first thought is vaginal delivery, followed by constipation,
> and ultimately Ehlers-Danlos syndrome and its variations. Pelvic
> organ prolapse and stress urinary incontinence in young nulliparous
> women can be a valuable finding in the diagnostic puzzle. Urogyne-
> cologists are sometimes the first doctors to encourage women to pursue
> further testing for connective tissue disorders. It is important to have
> a team of urogynecologist and colorectal surgeon when assessing and
> treating pelvic floor dysfunction in women with Ehlers-Danlos syn-
> drome."*
>
> Alexandra Dubinskaya, MD

EDS symptoms can vary considerably among patients, which does make diagnosis muddy. The POP/EDS intersect disrupts QOL in women as young as
mid-teens. Because there is a notable occurrence of POP within the young EDS
population, there is truly a need to enhance awareness to increase screening
and detection in young women. Girls with flexible joints are often enrolled in
gymnastics at a very young age. Given the nature of gymnastics often being a
childhood-long venture that includes hard foot strike activity (sticking gymnastic
landings), young athletes should be monitored for signs of pelvic floor weakness.
Urinary leakage is an indicator of pelvic floor weakness, a marker of EDS issues,
and flag of potential high risk of POP in the future.

Connective tissue manifestation within the hEDS community may include joint
hypermobility, skin hyperextensibility, fragile tissue, weak ligaments, hemorrhoids, hernias, digestive issues such as IBS, heartburn, or constipation, varicose
veins, soft velvety skin, diastasis rectus abdominus (DRA), intussusception, slow
wound healing, neuromuscular pain, and neuropathic pain. Additional indi-

cators of hEDS may including loose, unstable joints that dislocate easily, joint pain, clicking joints, extreme fatigue, skin that bruises easily, as well as dizziness and increased heart rate upon standing. POP and stress urinary incontinence (SUI) are common in hEDS women and may occur as young as teens years prior to pregnancy. Unique symptoms in young women are unquestionably a flag to screen for POP at an early age.

Women experiencing the POP/EDS overlap generally struggle to find a nonsurgical treatment to successfully relieve symptoms. They often struggle to capture long-term surgical success. They have a higher risk of surgical complications.

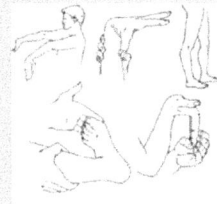

EDS/POP COMORBID CONDITION SYSTEM CHECK

EDS Screen	Beighton Score
➢ Digestive issues, IBS	
➢ Varicose veins	
➢ Hernia	
➢ Pain issues	
➢ Soft, velvety skin	
➢ POP/UI at young age	
➢ DRA, intussusception	
➢ Wounds slow to heal	
➢ Flexible joints	

Ehlers-Danlos Syndrome. Image courtesy of
Association for Pelvic Organ Prolapse Support.

Women with hEDS who have POP surgery have an increased risk of surgical failure, particularly with native tissue repair. Uterine prolapse incidence is common. Recurrent hernia is an hEDS screening marker. The rate of pain with intimacy in hEDS patients may be greater than in the general population, estimated to range between 30-61%, believed to be the impact of small tears in the vaginal wall and lack of appropriate vaginal secretions. Stress urinary incontinence was found in 40%–70% of women with hEDS, including frequent occurrences early in life associated with bladder prolapse. Fecal incontinence is estimated at 15% of hEDS patients, and rectal prolapse is more prevalent than in the general populace.

Women with hEDS have a higher risk of postpartum hemorrhage (19% versus 7%) and complicated perineal wounds (8% versus 0%).

Some of the surgical issues that may occur with POP treatment in the hEDS sector are higher rates of surgical failure in native tissue repair, mesh erosion, poor surgical wound healing, nerve entrapment, excess pain, wound reopening, birth trauma, extra stitches or use of steristrip reinforcement, plus additional time needed to heal before stitch removal. Women with hEDS often experience pain more severely, both a marker prior to and concern post-surgery. Joint and long-term widespread pain (greater than 3 months) are explicitly part of the criteria for diagnosis of hEDS.

Women experiencing collagen-associated disorders such as hEDS have an increased probability of prolapse severity, more acute POP symptoms, and a predisposition to polypropylene mesh erosion. Women experiencing the POP/EDS connection have the greatest difficulty capturing surgical success of all the diverse issues women with POP navigate.

Indicators of hEDS occur in multiple body systems and equally confuse practitioner and patient. Women commonly go through an extensive journey searching for an accurate analysis of their symptoms. Women with hEDS may experience considerable delay in diagnosis and are frequently misdiagnosed with fibromyalgia and chronic fatigue syndrome, are assumed to be hypochondriacs, and frequently experience depression at long-term lack of precise analysis. In the process of seeing multiple clinicians, women often have a sense of being demeaned and diminished while they continue to search for answers and effective treatment.

Inappropriate treatment can be a consequence. Two surveys involving 10,000 patients with 16 uncommon diseases indicated those with EDS experienced the most significant delay in diagnosis, with over half being misdiagnosed and 70% receiving improper treatment as a result.

There is no precise treatment for hEDS; patients are typically advised to avoid specific activities, particularly those related to heavy lifting, hard foot strike, or aggressive contact athletic activities. Low-risk fitness activities such as swimming or speed-walking are recommended to reduce probability of POP occurrence in general, but the significance of this is the POP/EDS sector is even more pronounced.

Symptoms of POP/EDS can be vague or obvious, are often multi-systemic, and are equally perplexing to patients and health care providers. Women with hEDS typically experience a long-term diagnostic journey, visiting multiple types of clinicians in different fields of practice looking for answers to diverse symptoms. Prior to receiving a correct diagnosis of EDS, women may experience frustration, dismissal, and belittlement and are often advised to seek psychiatric counseling for physical symptoms that are very real. The chase for EDS diagnosis may go on for years before the POP/EDS connection is recognized. Frequently EDS remains undiagnosed until surgical failure occurs multiple times.

Lifestyle and behavioral activities can compound the probability or degree of POP severity in the EDS patient. What is rarely recognized is the additional potential to impact post-surgical healing in the POP/EDS patient. Women are typically advised to return to normal activities 6 weeks post-surgery, once they have been cleared by examination. Women frequently do not feel healed at the 6-week point post POP surgery; at 8 weeks healing is further optimized. With complex or advanced POP surgeries, 12 weeks of healing may be necessary before returning to normal activities. The POP/EDS patient requires additional time, possibly an additional 3 months in more severe cases of hEDS, to ensure weak tissue has suitably healed before resuming normal activities.

While the physical struggles of women navigating POP/EDS are considerable, the frustrations they experience related to clinician dismissal are often pronounced and are usually intensified by experiencing it repetitively as they move from physician to physician. Patient voice nearly always clarifies health and health-care treatment reality. Following are the voices of women who have experienced POP/EDS navigation.

> *"I was diagnosed EDS because of chronic pelvic pain. They discovered I had stretch marks, keloids, paper-thin scars related to EDS. It impacts my ability to sit longer than a minute, do any sort of exercise as my SI joints are constantly inflamed. I'm still very toned, just quite weak in my lower half of the body. Employment was extremely difficult related to fatigue. Also standing for hours on end nursing caused a nasty flare in vaginismus and pelvic floor pain. The 'worst' for me is honestly the pain."*
>
> Age 43

> *"It isn't just ONE quality-of-life impact that is 'the worst'". The key is for doctors to really understand how devastating this is because it severely affects ALL areas of our lives. I had light-stress urine leakage*

my whole life and could never wear tampons, and my periods were agonizingly painful. I noticed the actual organs falling down was when I was 34 or 35. Full-on rapid prolapse at 35. The unrelenting pain which impacts emotional wellbeing, sexual interactions, the inability to maintain physical fitness, also made it impossible for me to continue working. Having a BM is now a constant source of distress... painful, embarrassing, constantly worrying about fecal incontinence so I basically stay home all the time, and of course worrying about leaking stool during sex is a total intimacy destroyer. The depression over the loss of self, the frequent doctor appointments and failed surgeries, the anger at my spouse for not making any effort to understand... The 'trigger stacking' with POP/EDS is enormous, the cumulative effect of how it impacts every aspect of our lives is overwhelming."

Age 47

"I've had eight POP-related surgeries since I gave birth to my daughter thirty years ago, but no one ever mentioned EDS to me."

Age 56

"There was no doubt to me that I had the hypermobile type of EDS (I also have velvet skin and other characteristics), and I asked my doctor to get a referral to the proper specialists. He laughed at me."

Age 45

"Could I have EDS? If yes, further surgery might be in vain. In fact, it might worsen things. Those were my thoughts based on the information from the internet. 'I guess you could have EDS,' my urogyn advised, 'but what do you want the diagnosis for? It doesn't make any difference.'"

Age 34

"10 years ago, at 35 I had my first symptoms, and my doctor knew I have hEDS, and brushed me off each time I mentioned my prolapse concerns and rectocele. She didn't offer any help or refer me to a urogynecologist until my uterus became a stage 3."

Age 45

"I was told I couldn't have POP before they even looked because I don't have kids. Then told I should just have kids because EDS will make my prolapse severe no matter what I do."

Age 27

"Diagnosed with EDS at 41 when I developed bladder, rectal, and uterine prolapse without ever having been pregnant. Went to "the best of the best" cash-pay surgeons because I was desperate for a good outcome. All of them said they had operated on many EDS patients. When I asked if they did anything differently during surgery because of EDS, like suture a distinct way, they said no and acted like I was stupid for worrying. Well, I've had ruptured internal sutures twice. After one of my operations, I told every doctor I saw for a year that all the symptoms I was dealing with came on in one day, exactly two months after said surgery. I expressed concern about my history with ruptured sutures. Every single time I was dismissed until I could actually see something protruding from my vagina again. Had another operation and low and behold, the sutures from my previous surgery had ruptured. In two words I would describe my last 3 years (4 operations) for prolapse as humiliation and dismissal!!"

Age 44

"I've had rectal prolapse since I was 19 or 20 and have never had kids. My first POP surgery was unsuccessful, and I had to have a second one a year ago with mesh (I am 26 now). So far it has been successful. No one mentioned EDS to me, my first surgeon said during surgery my collagen appeared "stretchy". I have some symptoms of connective tissue disorder but have never been diagnosed. Other than connective

tissue and constipation/disordered eating, I have no other explanation for the prolapse issues I will be struggling with for the rest of my life."

Age 26

To complicate the complexity of prolapse surgery, women with EDS often lack the tissue integrity to ensure repair will have long-term efficacy. POP procedures truly should be left to the experts, even more so in patients with POP/EDS co-existing conditions.

Every surgical procedure comes with risk, but surgical complications are rarely in patients' thoughts when they consult with physicians. Patients hope and expect their doctors to provide safe and appropriate care. Women with POP/EDS simply want their clinicians to listen to them, to believe them, to treat them with the same respect given to healthcare providers, even if they are sharing flies in the face of what their medical education has taught them.

18

LEVATOR AVULSION: THE MISSING LINK

APOPS Patient Perspective: *"I found my prolapse months into my post-partum journey, and immediately took a nosedive. My ob-gyn dismissed my anxiety as post-partum depression, when in reality is was high anxiety about having a deformed, dysfunctional body because sex is important to me and experiencing tissues bulging out of the vagina is horrifying. It would have been such a struggle to find ballast if I hadn't found APOPS amazing support structure."*
~PR, Rhode Island/USA

Women wonder why despite how frequently or well they perform Kegel exercises, their pelvic floor muscles never get stronger. Childbirth damage heals to varying degrees post-delivery in the months following birthing. However, some women with traumatic deliveries, particularly those involving forceps or suction delivery, may suffer long-term consequences of pelvic floor muscle damage.

Levator Avulsion (LA) occurs when part or all of the levator ani muscles rip off the pubic bone on one or both sides. These muscle defects increase both the risk and severity of pelvic organ prolapse since they reduce pelvic floor support. These injuries may also cause urinary or fecal continence.

The levator hiatus is the largest tissue opening in the human body.

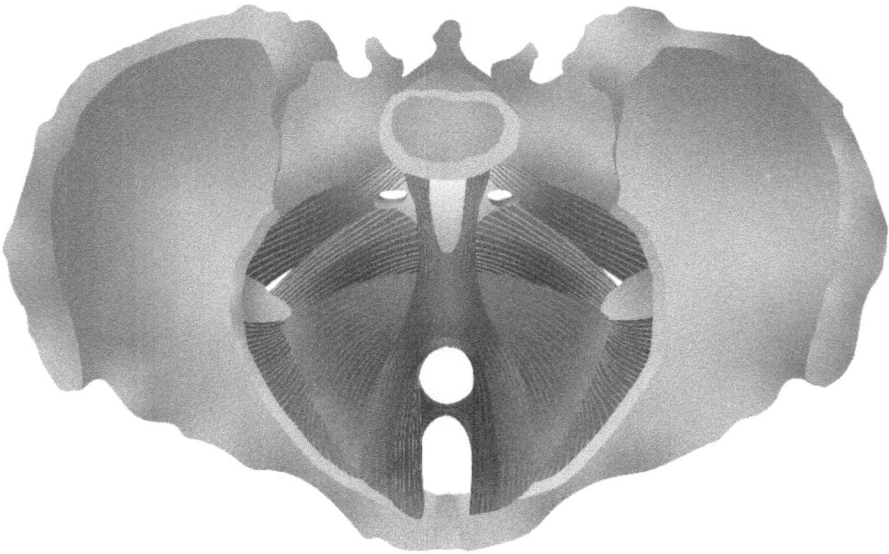

Levator Ani muscles. Image courtesy of
Association for Pelvic Organ Prolapse Support.

If the LA muscles have pulled off the pubic bones, the gap is wider. This increases the risk of organs pushing downward when intra-abdominal pressure occurs during heavy lifting, coughing, bending, or squatting. As indicated by the Birth Trauma Association, LA damage may result in:

- Increased LA muscle weakness by approximately 30%.

- Increased stretch of LA muscles by approximately 50%.

- Enlarged opening of the pelvic floor (hiatus) by approximately 25%.

- Doubled risk of bladder prolapse.

- Tripled risk of uterine prolapse.

- Tripled risk of a prolapse returning post pelvic floor surgery.

Evolution of 3D/4D ultrasound & MRI imagery in the pelvic floor space has led to an advanced understanding of LA issues by a very select number of specialists within the POP space. A urogynecologist and a women's health physical therapist far ahead of the curve in the LA space responded to questions submitted by women who have experienced LA damage.

S. Abbas Shobeiri, MD, MBA, is the INOVA Health System Chief of Benign Gynecology, a professor of Obstetrics and Gynecology Medical Education, and an affiliate biomedical engineering faculty at George Mason University. Dr. Shobeiri is an international authority in pelvic floor ultrasonography medical device development and pelvic floor ultrasonography, and a global expert in levator avulsion. Here is what Dr. Shobeiri had to share.

· · · · ●· ● ● ·· ·

THE BASICS:

Q. CLARIFY THE CAUSES OF LEVATOR ANI MUSCLE INJURY (LAMI).

"The best-known risk factors are forceps deliveries. Other than that we have seen LAM injuries with some of the most ordinary vaginal deliveries."

Q. WHAT ARE SYMPTOMS OF LAMI?

"Depending on the site of injury and severity, the symptoms can be different ranging from pressure with standing, feeling of vaginal bulge, vaginal gaping, to leakage of urine or stool, or inability to evacuate urine or stool. Some women report vaginal pain and also lack of or reduced ability to have sexual interest or orgasm."

Q. IS THERE A WAY TO AVOID LAMI?

"We advocate self-stretching of the LAM starting at 36 weeks. Also, a controlled confident vaginal birth is very important. It cannot be too slow with over 3 hours of active pushing or too rapid."

Q. HOW COMMON IS LAMI?

"Severe cases account for about 11-13% of all vaginal births. But hematomas (blood clots) in torn levator ani muscles can be detected in 39% of first and 11% of subsequent vaginal births."

Q. HOW IS POSTPARTUM LAMI DIAGNOSED?

"The diagnosis starts with realizing that the symptoms are abnormal and not consistent with normal resolution of vaginal delivery symptoms. Physical examination by a skilled practitioner is a must. In a recent study of women who were seen in our "motheRs' pElviC flOor sUpPort (RECOUP) Clinic", more than 50% were self-referred after seeing more than two practitioners. Also, frequently they were referred to us by our vast network of pelvic floor therapists. At the RECOUP clinic, the patients undergo a 3D endovaginal ultrasound which takes literally five minutes to complete. The process is very efficient to maximize our time with the patients to educate them about their specific injury and attend to their psychological needs as well. The pelvic floor anatomy which includes the LAM anatomy is complex. Most patients are in various stages of postpartum post-traumatic stress disorder (P-PTSD) which requires dedicated time and resources for psychological assessment and follow-up.

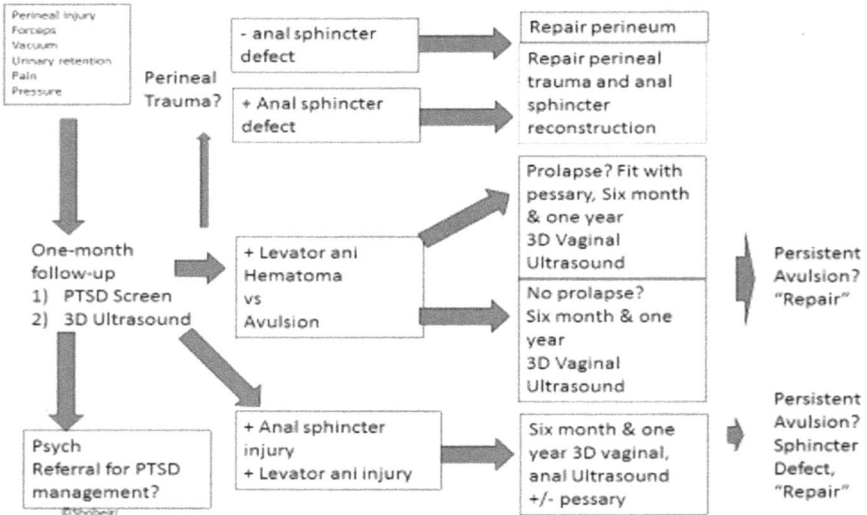

Levator avulsion diagnosis. Image courtesy of
Abbas Shobeiri, MD.

The patients are frequently relieved to know there is an organic cause for how they feel as less skilled providers may tell them nothing is wrong with them, or the family may create demands on them, and neither the patient nor the family understands the cause of her symptoms. They just know something is wrong and since the healthcare practitioners cannot find anything wrong, they conclude that it must be all in the patient's head. Confirming the diagnosis with the best imaging modality available is the first step on the long road to recovery."

Clinical Indications for 3D Endovaginal US

Signs & Symptoms

Anal Incontinence

Obstructed defecation

Voiding dysfunction

Pelvic pain and dyspareunia

Levator ani deficiency/pelvic floor muscle wasting

Pelvic organ prolapse

Perineal cyst or mass

Urethral hypermobility associated with UI

Vaginal cyst or mass such as urethral diverticulum

Post-partum assessment

Levator ani muscle assessment after childbirth

Obstetric perineal injury

Obstetric Anal Sphincter Injury

Post-surgical assessment

Pelvic or vaginal pain after synthetic implants (meshes or bulking agents)

Vaginal discharge or bleeding after pelvic floor surgery

3-D ultrasound indicators. Image courtesy of
Abbas Shobeiri, MD.

· · · ● · ● · ● · · ·

PATIENT QUESTIONS:

Q. WHAT MAKES LA UNFIXABLE?

"The levator ani muscle (LAM) is fixable. The LAM has a wide attachment to the pelvic side wall structures. Some portions of the pubococcygeus and puborectalis also have connections to the pubic bone. The LAM tissue can visually be compared to a trampoline. The trampoline attaches to the pelvic side wall and also to the sides of the pubic bones. We don't use the term levator avulsion as it is loosely used. Using endovaginal ultrasound, we find exactly where the muscle is injured. Compare it with a few of the springs holding the trampoline to the metal ring with various ways of the attachments having the possibility of injury. 3D perineal ultrasound is generally too nonspecific on the location of the injury because the bone obscures the muscles behind it with a shadow. 3D Endovaginal ultrasound overcomes this

limitation.

In other muscles in our body such as the calf muscle, we see that after damaging the Achilles tendon, the muscle roles up and is completely dysfunctional. In the LAM, we see that the function of the trampoline (supporting the organs) and its constricting and lifting capacity is decreased and sometimes totally gone. The muscle still stays in place, still doing its job, but at a lesser capacity."

Q. WHAT ARE POTENTIAL NEW WAYS TO ADDRESS LAMI?

"Research has looked at supporting the levator hiatus (the u-shaped gap in tissue at the front of the levator ani) with mesh with disastrous results. But they are also exploring the use of pessaries to replace the support of the levator at surgeries to reattach the muscle. The use of stem cells to "seed and grow" new muscular fibers and cure the damaged parts is still very early. Currently, my practice is like that of an orthopedist where I look at the individual's 3D endovaginal ultrasound and tactically directly repair various sites of injury with stitches regardless of if they are muscles, ligaments, or connective tissue. For a surgeon to perform these surgeries successfully they need to attain core competency in 3D endovaginal ultrasound and expertise in advanced deep tissue surgical techniques. We hope to publish our results and outcomes for the last three years in the near future."

Q. ARE POP SYMPTOMS WITH AND WITHOUT LAMI DIFFERENT?

"Yes, LAMi may cause more pronounced symptoms, such as a dragging and heavy feeling. Also, the risk of developing a significant prolapse is higher. The side that is not injured pulls and goes into spasm to compensate. So, during our repairs of one sides LAMi it is not uncommon to inject Botox in the intact LAM to relax it."

Q. WHY DON'T WOMEN'S HEALTH PRACTITIONERS SCREEN FOR LAM WHEN DIAGNOSING PROLAPSE (INSTEAD OF POP-Q EXAM ALONE CONFIRMING THE PROLAPSE)?

"Immediately after delivery, the woman is sore and uncertain what to expect. With LAM hiatus having to dilate during vaginal birth to three times its normal size, most women have some degree of LAMi that may heal spontaneously. If there is prolapse, severe pain, fecal or urinary incontinence, or third or fourth-degree lacerations, we ask for the patients to be referred to our RECOUP clinic for evaluation. Even a month after delivery, there are hematomas throughout the pelvis. We perform 3D endovaginal ultrasound at presentation and then at 6 months and

one year. If at one year, the woman still has evidence of prolapse and injury on 3D endovaginal ultrasound, and they are finished with childbearing, we offer them LAM repair. Meanwhile they are supported by psychological help AND pessary, hormones, and/or directed pelvic floor therapy depending on their injury."

Q. WHAT TYPE/STYLE OF PESSARY SEEMS TO WORK BEST?

"We seem to mostly use a ring pessary with or without support. Anything else can be painful postpartum especially if the patient is breastfeeding."

Q. WHAT IS THE DIFFERENCE BETWEEN A COMPLETE AND PARTIAL AVULSION, EITHER UNILATERAL OR BILATERAL. WHICH MUSCLES ARE USUALLY INVOLVED?

"We don't use terms complete or partial as 3D endovaginal ultrasound is very specific on what is injured. The levator ani muscle is not a single muscle. It is composed of puboperinealis, puboanalis, puborectalis, pubococcygeus, and iliococcygeus muscles, one on either side of the pelvis. The most commonly injured muscle is the pubococcygeus and since it is next to the iliococcygeus, it opens up like a zipper from the side wall, causing the prolapse of the bladder on the injured side. Most often the right-side muscles are injured as the rectum gives some degree of protection to the left side."

Q. WHAT IMPACT DOES LAMI HAVE ON A SUBSEQUENT VAGINAL BIRTH?

"It was thought that the first vaginal birth caused all the damage, but our research has shown that there is continued injury to the muscles with subsequent vaginal births. Also, pregnancy alone has an adverse effect on the pelvic floor due to the hormonal changes that occur since progesterone loosens the ligaments in the pelvis."

Q. DOES HAVING LAMI PREDICT POORER POP SURGICAL OUTCOMES?

"Depending on the surgery and depending on the kind of injuries sustained, different surgeries can be employed. LAMi that is postpartum may be repaired at the time of prolapse surgery. The LAM in reality is perhaps ½ the equation. When the fascial defects are repaired only ½ the equation is solved."

Q. WHAT IS THE GOLD STANDARD FOR RECOVERY PLAN AFTER LAMI?

"The first step is diagnosis that the injury has occurred, and to do this accurately imaging is required. Once injury is confirmed, the immediate recovery is like any other muscle. RICE stands for rest, ice, compression, and elevation, and taking these simple steps following a strain, sprain, or other similar injury can help the patients to recover more quickly and get back to everyday activities. For the pelvic floor we advocate Rest, Ice, Pessary, and Constipation control."

Q. IS THE LEVATOR ANI AFFECTED PERMANENTLY TO SOME DEGREE IN ALL VAGINAL BIRTHS?

"Our studies have shown that 39% of women first-time mothers and 11% of subsequent mothers who deliver vaginally have hematomas at the site of injury to their LAM."

Q. MY DOCTOR SAYS LEVATOR AVULSION CAN ONLY BE DETECTED VIA MRI. MY PELVIC FLOOR THERAPIST SAID SHE COULD TELL; SHE FELT AROUND AND SAID I DIDN'T HAVE ONE. WHO SHOULD I BELIEVE?

"Only the most severe varieties may be diagnosed with palpation. Once suspected, it needs to be confirmed with 3D endovaginal ultrasound, MRI, or 3D perineal ultrasound, although the latter is probably best for avulsion diagnosis."

· · · · **·** · **·** · · · ·

Hedwig Neels MScPT, PhD is a pelvic floor and women's health physiotherapist. She currently is a postdoc research assistant at the University of Antwerp, Faculty of Medicine and Health Care, within MOVANT & ASTARC, expanding expertise in pelvic floor assessments with 3D/4D transperineal ultrasound.

Q. WHAT MAKES LA UNFIXABLE?

"The levator ani is probably one of the only muscles in our body that has a direct attachment of muscular tissue to bony tissue. Most of our muscles attach to the bone via a tendon. The levator ani muscular tissue can visually be compared to a

trampoline. The trampoline attaches to the sides of the pelvic bones. Luckily, in case of levator avulsion, we often see that only parts of the attachment are damaged. Compare it with a few of the ropes tying the trampoline to the metal stand with most of the ropes loose but still attached. Most of the trampoline would remain in place.

"The levator ani is probably one of the only muscles in our body that has a direct attachment of muscular tissue to bony tissue. Most of our muscles attach to the bone via a tendon. The levator ani muscular tissue can visually be compared to a trampoline. The trampoline attaches to the sides of the pelvic bones. Luckily, in case of levator avulsion, we often see that only parts of the attachment are damaged. Compare it with a few of the ropes tying the trampoline to the metal stand with most of the ropes loose but still attached. Most of the trampoline would remain in place.

In other muscles in our body such as the calf muscle, if the Achilles tendon is torn, the muscle roles up and is completely dysfunctional. In the levator, we see that the function of the trampoline (supporting the organs) and its constricting and lifting capacity is decreased, but it is not gone. The muscle still remains in position doing its job, but at a lesser capacity."

Q. WHAT ARE POTENTIAL NEW WAYS TO ADDRESS LEVATOR AVULSION?

"Research is looking at supporting the levator hiatus (the u-shaped gap in tissue at the front of the levator ani) with mesh. But they are also exploring the use of pessaries to replace the support of the levator, at surgeries to reattach the muscle, and stem cells to "seed and grow" new muscular fibers and cure the damaged parts. But on the current time the success ratio remains low."

Q. ARE POP SYMPTOMS WITH AND WITHOUT AVULSION DIFFERENT?

"Yes, levator avulsion causes more pronounced symptoms, such as a dragging and heavy feeling. Also, the risk of developing a significant prolapse is higher. Clinically, I also often see that in some women with unilateral (one-sided) avulsion, the opposite side seems to compensate with a tendency to be hypertonic (tight muscle tone). Often, I notice women have a tender and painful zone in the "intact" side. But to the best of my knowledge, that is not yet confirmed in research data."

Q. WHY DON'T WOMEN'S HEALTH PRACTITIONERS SCREEN FOR LA WHEN DIAGNOSING PROLAPSE (INSTEAD OF POP-Q EXAM ALONE CONFIRMING THE PROLAPSE)?

"I think that it's extremely important to also screen for levator ani avulsion. We know that LA increases the risk of developing significant prolapse, so prevention becomes even more critical. Also, lifestyle tips such as avoiding constipation should be emphasized. But even more important, we know that levator avulsion decreases the muscle force and endurance. If women have partial or complete avulsion at both sides, they often have less capacity to constrict and perform a Kegel contraction. If they are not informed about this, they get disappointed in the results that they get with exercises. They often feel guilty for not getting results in exercise therapy. They often feel like they are doing something wrong if trainers are not detecting what is not functioning properly.

Therefore we need to screen to raise awareness, to reassure women that we understand their problems, to help them understand that they can benefit from training their muscles!"

Q. WHAT TYPE/STYLE OF PESSARIES SEEM TO WORK BEST?

"Really varies from woman to woman."

Q. WHAT IS THE DIFFERENCE BETWEEN A COMPLETE AND PARTIAL AVULSION, EITHER UNILATERAL OR BILATERAL. WHICH MUSCLES ARE USUALLY INVOLVED?

"The levator ani muscle is a V-shaped muscled. I compared it before with a trampoline, but that is to explain what this muscle does. It actually is a hammock shape that is attached quite high in the pelvis. This means that instead of comparing the pelvic floor with a bowl, we should compare it to a funnel, with a V or U-shaped hiatus gap in the middle, to allow the urethra, vagina, and anal canal passage, with attachments of the muscle at both sides of the symphysis pubis between the pubic bones. If one side of the V is damaged, we call it a unilateral avulsion; if both sides are avulsed, it is a bilateral avulsion."

Q. WHAT IMPACT DOES LA HAVE ON A SUBSEQUENT VAGINAL BIRTH?

"Often the subsequent vaginal birth will not cause further damage to the avulsion itself, but it might worsen a prolapse."

Q. DOES HAVING AVULSION PREDICT POORER POP SURGICAL OUTCOMES?

"Yes."

Q. WHAT IS THE GOLD STANDARD FOR RECOVERY PLAN?

"Firstline treatment guidelines promote pelvic floor muscle training. But it might be more difficult or even in some women impossible to reach the same results as in those without avulsion."

Q. IS THE LEVATOR ANI AFFECTED PERMANENTLY TO SOME DEGREE IN ALL VAGINAL BIRTHS?

"No, from a study of Jessica Caudwell Hall (What do women really want?) we see that in +/- 33% no avulsion or no remaining hiatal ballooning or overdistention is detected. So at least one out of three women has no damage."

Q. MY DOCTOR SAYS LEVATOR AVULSION CAN ONLY BE DETECTED VIA MRI. MY PELVIC FLOOR THERAPIST SAID SHE COULD TELL; SHE FELT AROUND AND SAID I DIDN'T HAVE ONE. WHO SHOULD I BELIEVE?

"Detection can be done with MRI or transperineal ultrasound, but indeed also with vaginal palpation."

· · · · ● · ● · · ·

In today's society, many women are tuned into fitness. Others recognize notable changes in their pelvic floor post-childbirth. Regardless the personal dynamic, when women are frantically working away at their pelvic floor strength and experience little improvement of symptoms, they become frustrated without knowing the why.

Levator ani avulsion has puzzled the medical community for a long time, with whispers of concerns dating back to midwifery in 1808. Research is critical to capture a greater understanding in this significant aspect of the pelvic floor puzzle. As expansion of imaging techniques enhances exploration, women wondering how and why their bodies are misbehaving will gain hope.

19

FECAL INCONTINENCE: NEXT STEPS WHEN YOUR BODY ROADBLOCKS ROMANCE

APOPS Patient Perspective: "Because of APOPS and the sharing of experiences in their group, my shame, despair, and fear turned into confidence and hope."

~DD, UK

One of the most highly stigmatizing POP symptoms is fecal incontinence (FI). Regardless of when FI occurs it is devastating, but if it occurs during an act of intimacy, the impact is difficult to move past. The fear of a repeat episode, the anxiety of judgment by an intimate partner, and the apprehension of never again having a normal sex life can create a significant roadblock in a woman's life.

"The impact of prolapse on the health and well-being of women, and especially older women, is sadly neglected and under-appreciated. Unfortunately, the shame, embarrassment, and stigma of fecal incontinence make seeking care less likely despite the many available treatment options. Clinicians really need to ensure that they proactively and sensitively inquire about these conditions at every routine opportunity."

Adrian Wagg, MD

Fecal incontinence is one of those POP symptoms women struggle to admit to, much less talk about openly. But as in all aspects of POP, it is possible to find your way back to balance once you discover a relatively comfortable path to talk about FI and the appropriate tools to address it. A brave patient in APOPS' following agreed to share her journey in the interest of providing hope for others walking this particular walk.

· · · ● · ● · ● · · ·

Q. WHERE WERE YOU IN YOUR POP JOURNEY WHEN FECAL IN-CONTINENCE OCCURRED? WERE YOU NEWLY DIAGNOSED, OR HAD YOU ALREADY BEEN TREATED FOR POP WITH NON-SURGI-CAL OR SURGICAL TREATMENTS?

I had been diagnosed at 24 with rectocele (grade 3), cystocele grade 2, and slight uterine prolapse (I am assuming grade 1). At 27, I had a full hysterectomy (related to cervical issues), along with a rectocele repair, sacrospinous ligament fixation, and perineoplasty. I had some fecal incontinence prior to the surgery (maybe twice I can recall) and several times after my surgery.

Q. HOW DEVASTATING DID YOU INITIALLY FIND THE DIAGNOSIS OF POP AND WERE YOU IN A RELATIVELY BALANCED EMOTION-AL STATE OF MIND REGARDING THIS CONDITION WHEN FECAL INCONTINENCE OCCURRED?

I was more shocked at first. I thought it was so embarrassing, but I began working in women's health about 4 months after my initial diagnosis and began educating myself. Being a nurse, I've been very open with pretty much anyone willing to listen. I wasn't as bothered by the fecal incontinence emotionally because it didn't happen immediately, and it wasn't often. I guess I was at a good place with it. Talking about fecal incontinence has been my coping mechanism with it.

Q. HOW OLD WERE YOU WHEN YOU FIRST EXPERIENCED FECAL INCONTINENCE DURING AN ACT OF INTIMACY?

I was 28 and about 10 months post-surgery.

Q. WHAT EXACTLY OCCURRED DURING YOUR FI EPISODE?

It occurred during climax, and I had no idea it had happened until my partner noticed.

Q. HOW DID YOUR PARTNER REACT, WAS HE FREAKED OUT, DID HE LAUGH IT OFF, SHRUG IT OFF, NOT REACT AT ALL?

He was great about it. At first, he laughed it off, but when he saw I was devastated, he assured me it wasn't a big deal. And continues to do so the few times we've talked about it. I cried in the shower afterwards. The days following, I was so depressed. The day after, I cried pretty much on and off all day.

Q. WHAT ANXIETY DO YOU HAVE ABOUT FI OCCURRING AGAIN DURING INTIMACY?

I've been intimate once since and I have to say I am terrified it will happen again. The stress did impact my ability to climax; I was unable to relax to enjoy intimacy and I felt very emotional afterwards.

Q. WHAT STEPS DID YOU/WILL YOU TAKE TO PREVENT A REPEAT EPISODE?

I make sure to go to the bathroom before. I did sort of schedule sex (our schedules kind of roadblock us sometimes).

Q. DID YOU HAVE AN OPEN CONVERSATION WITH YOUR INTIMATE PARTNER ABOUT WHAT OCCURRED?

Yes. I explained no matter how supportive he has been; this is still my huge struggle. I think this was the straw that broke the camel's back for my feelings towards intimacy post-surgery. It's been a process of recovery and I'm still not there yet. I start another round of physical therapy next week (I wasn't great about going after my 6-week appointment because of scheduling conflicts and childcare). I am sure I place excess emphasis on this event, and I have conflicting feelings towards how my body has changed after surgery. I also have thick permanent surgical sutures that have been impacting intimacy. But simply talking about it helps me cope.

· · · · ●·● · · · ·

Obviously, women react differently to experiencing FI. Here are a few things to consider:

- Fecal incontinence is usually a much bigger deal to the women who experience it than it is to their intimate partners. The endgame is at times satisfying partners sexually, and anything else occurring is not even on the radar.

- Post-surgery, nerves take longest to heal, up to a year. If you are experiencing FI, contact your surgeon and ask for input. Your surgeon is familiar with your pelvic particulars and may be able to shine a bit of light on next steps from the medical perspective. In general, behavior modification can be a priceless tool. Moving forward, experiment with techniques to reduce the possibility of FI occurring.

- Pay attention to what you eat prior to intimacy. This is a good idea in general, even if there aren't FI issues. There's nothing like releasing a blast of gas during an act of intimacy to make women squirm. Avoid foods that will increase likelihood of digestive issues.

- Pay attention to the state of your "guts" prior to intimacy. If you have had a stressful day or ate a half hour prior to intimacy, it increases the risk of FI in those who experience it.

- Pay attention to what position you take during intimacy. Experiment with a variety of positions with female on the bottom or side. Avoid being on top.

Moving forward: humor is your best friend. We women clean up baby poop, puppy poop, cat poop, parent poop and don't think twice about it other than dealing with smell or mess in the moment. But if incontinence happens to us, we are totally freaked out. Everyone comes into this world pooping in their pants and most of us will go out the same way. We really need to get past anxiety about leakage regardless what type it is or orifice it comes out of. Being able to joke comfortably about FI takes a bit of time, but humor is incredibly healing.

A woman is going to be extremely nervous about the first attempt at intimacy after an episode of FI. Take it slow. Talk to your partner about your anxiety while sharing a glass of wine or cup of tea to relax. And if you are too nervous to give it a go in your bed, maybe it's time to experiment with shower sex.

20

IMPACT TO INTIMACY

APOPS Patient Perspective: "At the age of 27, I felt like I was trapped inside the body of an 80-year-old woman, but the empathy, understanding, and guidance I received from the other women in APOPS forum provided a path back to balance that even my doctor could not provide."

~AT, Minnesota/USA

With nearly every topic discussed blatantly these days in media, most health issues land squarely out in the open. Conversations related to sexual energy are generally considered acceptable topics of conversation. Unfortunately, the stigmatizing symptoms of POP hinder dialogue about this extremely common women's health condition.

The aspect of POP that I get the strongest reaction to when connecting with women in APOPS patient support forum, speaking at conferences or public events, or while being interviewed by the media, is the impact of POP to intimacy. Coital incontinence (leakage of urine or stool during acts of intimacy), overactive bladder, the awkward visual of tissues bulging from the vagina, large vaginal gap reducing sensation, chronic constipation, vaginal or rectal pressure, lack of sexual sensation, inability to orgasm, or back or pelvic pain, can roadblock a pleasurable sexual experience, and at times turn it into a problematic intimate event. As a result, women understandably at times avoid intimate relations. The ripple effect to relationships can be overwhelming.

The physical act of intimacy is a pivotal facet of a close connection with our partners. Without physical intimacy, some women emotionally disconnect from the relationship bond. Awareness of a pelvic health issue that needs to be addressed may help intimate partners recognize that it is not for lack of wanting intimacy that women hold back - it is a matter of discomfort, embarrassment, or both. Treatment often helps intimate partners reconnect.

Thanks to the breast cancer campaigns of Komen and National Breast Cancer Foundation in the 1980s, breast cancer stigma came to a halt. Prior to that, few spoke about breast cancer out loud; the word breast was not allowed in printed publications such as newspapers or magazines, and breast conversations were considered "off the table". We now recognize and freely talk about breast health. We created a comfort zone with awareness.

In 1998, few spoke about erectile dysfunction (ED) out loud prior to Pfizer providing a beacon of hope for men with the little blue pill. We now openly see ED pharmaceutical commercials during prime-time television and ads in magazines, men freely admit to using the little blue pill and women are perfectly ok with that. Hundreds of thousands of men are treated for ED annually, and everyone speaks comfortably about ED. We created a comfort zone with awareness.

Thanks to the media and some savvy ad campaigns, stigma has been removed from both breast cancer and ED. We need to get to the page where we speak freely about POP and all of the symptoms, including those that impact intimacy.

While women with pelvic organ prolapse navigate physical, emotional, social, sexual, fitness, and employment quality of life impact, intimacy is a zone that continues to carry the most significant baggage. Generally, we women talk about pretty much everything. We freely give up gory details about childbirth.

They told me to push and then next thing you know, I pooped on the table.

My water broke in the middle of the mall; the guy walking next to me almost threw up.

The intern had his hand up inside of me b/4 he even introduced himself.

You get the picture.

So how exactly does POP cause issues in the bedroom? Typically, women with POP can experience numerous symptoms that may interfere with the intimacy they emotionally covet but find physically unfeasible.

- Vaginal tissue bulge. Without a doubt the most common symptom of

POP, women who feel vaginal pressure or tissues bulging when they wipe after urinating may take a look with a mirror to see what is going on down below. Most often, what appears to be a tumor coming out of your vagina prompts a visit to the gynecologist, after which POP may be diagnosed. From that point forward, women often feel their nether regions look unattractive to men and shut down the gates.

- Vaginal pressure. Intercourse may feel like trying to stuff the toothpaste back in the tube because tissues and the organs behind them bulge into the vagina, shrinking vaginal space.

- Pain. Often women with POP experience vaginal, rectal, abdominal, or back pain. For some, pain with intercourse prevents intimacy altogether, no matter what sexual position. Women try to explain to their partners what the pain is like, but it is extremely difficult to put words to pelvic discomfort related to POP. Women may not be believed by the men in their lives when expressing that pain holds them back. While what I experienced wasn't pain, I used to say it felt like someone turned an electric mixer on in my guts. Some women are able to distinguish POP pain as sharp, dull, an ache, pulling, others not. Since there are five types of POP and four levels of severity with many combinations of POP types; pain is very individual.

- Chronic constipation. Chronic constipation is the status quo when it comes to rectocele. Chronic constipation can lead to persistent bloat, that stuffed sausage sensation. Not the type of occasional irregular-ity that Activia talks about, more like I haven't pooped more than raisin-sized stool in a week, and I'd hand over my first-born child to have one-normal-bowel-movement type of constipation. Discomfort ranges from mild to excruciating. Constipation once in a while is tolerable; on a daily basis it is enough to make an ogre out of an angel. All you want to do is have one good poop. And the last thing you want is more "stuff" inside of you-needless to say, adding a penis to the clutter causing pressure inside the pelvic cavity can be a bit distressing.

- Urine retention. The flip side of incontinence is urine retention, which is common in higher grades 3 and 4 of POP severity, and is what I experienced. No matter how badly I had to pee, urine was simply not coming out. Picture a garden hose crimped in half stopping the flow of water-that was my urethra. Now imagine a penis blasting into your full bladder over and over.

- Coital incontinence (CI). Yes, it is exactly what it sounds like. During the physical engagement of intimacy, urine or stool leaks out of your body. It's nearly impossible to share such personal information with a partner ahead of the curve. Loss of urine or stool in day-to-day activities is one thing, but how on earth do you handle leakage in the middle of an intimate act? Talk about a mood breaker. CI occurs relatively frequently, but women underreport CI occurrence either because they don't realize they are leaking urine or they are too embarrassed to share this detail with anyone. A 2018 international study of 1041 women in the Journal of Sexual Medicine indicated 53.8% of women in the study experienced coital urinary incontinence (CUI): 8% at penetration, 35% during intercourse, 9% at orgasm, and 48% during a combination of these sexual actions. While fecal incontinence also occurs, it is rarely reported by patients.

- Lack of intimate sensation. Women may experience a lack of clitoral sensation. Women who used to be capable of coming to an orgasm relatively easily find it a bit disillusioning to lose sensation altogether. Many very busy women feel as though they might as well get the kitchen cleaned up if they aren't experiencing physical or emotional satisfaction.

What will it take to break the silence? Vaginal health is health and sexual health is health. Talking about POP and all the symptoms out loud will evolve awareness, diagnostics, support, and screening, pivotal to shift women's pelvic health dynamic forward.

Women unfamiliar with pelvic organ prolapse typically have no idea that embarrassing or debilitating symptoms they experience during acts of intimacy might be related to POP. Many women struggle to find ballast with no idea how. As with other areas of the POP dynamic, women dealing with the POP impact to intimacy need to know they are not alone and that there is help available.

"POP is a health concern which connotes almost a "taboo-like" quality related to both interpersonal as well as professional communication, and one that is surrounded by substantial gaps of knowledge and inherently wrong information, much of it imparted by well-meaning but incompletely informed sources."

Roger Dmochowski, MD

Over the years as I have engaged in POP advocacy, thousands of women have come forward with intimacy concerns. Some were looking for emotional support, or dumping baggage, or searching for the specialists who treat POP, or simply looking for basic POP info. Multiple common themes emerged. These women were angry that they were not informed about POP until after they were diagnosed. Many were fearful of losing their husbands or boyfriends because having sex was painful and their partners didn't understand their pain or believe them.

D was extremely distraught when she first approached me; her life had completely unraveled before she was able to figure out what was happening to her body. At the age of 45, she was newly divorced. The prior four years she'd had significant pain while engaging in intercourse. While she also had ongoing problems with stomach bloat and distention, the multiple tests her physician ran all came back negative and he recommended she consider utilizing anti-anxiety medications. D did not want to take medications that would alter her state of mind, she was still raising two teenagers and wanted to be as clear-headed as possible to address their needs. Her relationship with her husband started to deteriorate because intercourse became so painful she started to find excuses to avoid it. She tried to explain to her husband it hurt to have sex. Initially he believed her, but eventually he became quite disgruntled. After a period of time, he stopped attempting intimacy. He started working late at night and going to the office on the weekend.

When her husband asked for a divorce, D was devastated. How on earth was she supposed to pick up the pieces of her life and start a new relationship when intimacy was painful? D felt like damaged goods that no man would want. It was difficult enough meeting someone new; how on earth could she explain to someone of the opposite sex that intercourse is painful? Fortunately, the change in her insurance coverage related to her divorce led to a new gynecologist who diagnosed D's symptoms as pelvic organ prolapse. Once she was referred to a subspecialist and diagnosed with a grade 3 rectocele and cystocele, she went online looking for answers and found APOPS support forum. Being able to share her story with other women helped her get through the steps she needed to make treatment decisions as well as helped her gain the confidence to move on with her personal life.

N experienced coital incontinence. She was not aware that coital incontinence was "a thing"; all she knew was every time she attempted to be intimate with her partner, she leaked urine. The day she leaked stool, sex was over for her. She found it unbearable to be intimate for fear of a repeat episode. She could not bring herself to disclose the issue to her physician, and she couldn't bear the thought of asking other women about her symptoms. She suffered in silence as often occurs.

Fortunately for N, her husband loved her greatly and kept prodding her about the reasons for lack of intimacy and encouraged her to speak with her physician, which led to a POP diagnosis and treatment.

T was a young woman in her 20s who experienced traumatic forceps delivery along with considerable damage to her pelvic floor. She never recovered from the birth trauma, and within months of her delivery, noticed tissues bulging out of her vagina. Horrified her husband would see them and be turned off, she also started refusing intimacy and figured her sex life was over. Luckily for T, someone in her inner circle who was also experiencing pelvic organ prolapse shared that information and this empowered T to start asking questions and digging online for information.

IMPACT TO INTIMACY – Patient Voice

"The gaping visual effect."

"Complete loss of sensation."

"Bathroom urge as soon as we start which gets worse as we continue."

"Always feeling kind of moist."

"Fear of stool loss."

"Pain from dryness."

"The betrayal of your body goes to the very core of your sexuality."

Pelvic organ prolapse impact to intimacy. Image courtesy of Association for Pelvic Organ Prolapse Support.

All the women I have mentioned had a very basic concern in common - none of them knew about pelvic organ prolapse prior to being diagnosed.

None of them recognized POP symptoms.

None of them knew POP causes.

None of them knew measures they should be taking to address POP symptoms or quality of life impacts.

None of them knew where to get information because so little open dialogue about POP occurs.

As pelvic organ prolapse awareness expands, conversations about POP will normalize. As the medical community expands screening to an appropriate level, stigma will fade. In the enlightened POP reality, women won't be afraid to initiate a conversation to capture the information they need.

21

POP MISCONCEPTIONS

APOPS Patient Perspective: *"APOPS enlightened me with a wealth of treatment insights, self-help suggestions, and diverse information no doctor would have or take the time to share. I no longer feel alone in this journey."*

~AD, Oregon/USA

I f you want to know the reality of any health condition, ask the patient. When it comes to a condition shrouded in silence such as POP, multiply the confusion substantially.

There are a multitude of misconceptions about POP. The most common misconception is likely prevalence. Does POP occur in 3% of women? 10%? 40%? Research routinely indicates up to 50% of the female population experiences POP. The reality is we won't have accurate prevalence numbers until POP screening becomes a standardized aspect of routine pelvic exams.

Let's explore patient voice regarding misconceptions in this women's healthcare space. The misconceptions shared below are comments from women walking the POP walk within the APOPS patient support structure.

"My first surgeon told me 'all will be as it was before you had children.' Not true. Never was, never will be."

"POP isn't a big deal because it's not life-threatening."

"That you just need to do more kegels."

"POP isn't painful. BS!"

"Low-grade prolapses don't cause any symptoms."

"That POP is "normal" after bearing children. (Common yes, normal NO!)"

"We are led to believe that successful POP surgery is when all the organs are 'back in place', rather than when the woman has a return to pre-POP quality of life."

"No woman who is a fit for surgery will consider colpocleisis unless she is very, very old."

"That pessaries are for older women."

"Patronizingly being told by physician he can see the bulge, but to not worry, nothing needs to be done."

"It's normal for women to pee when they laugh, jump, etc."

"That young women can't have POP!"

"That your life is over. We have options!"

"That we women don't know what we are feeling or talking about when we go to the doctor with POP issues. Grrrr."

"That everyone with POP pees in their pants. (Some do, I didn't.)"

"That young women can't wear a pessary!"

"That you need to be fixed in order to improve sex for your partner."

"You're too young for POP surgery."

"That it is JUST a 'quality of life' issue. The last time I checked, quality of life was hugely important!"

"Surgery is a quick fix; 6 weeks and good as new!"

"That PT won't help if prolapse is too advanced."

"That pelvic floor dysfunction is always about loose muscles, but sometimes the pelvic floor muscles are too tight."

"The cure prescribed for POP constipation is exercise and high fiber diet, but many of us find that high fiber supplements make it worse."

"I think the biggest misconception I came across was from my primary care GP who examined me and literally said, "you don't have prolapse". I felt gaslighted and ashamed that what I was experiencing didn't exist. In fact, I had multiple prolapses and needed repair and a pelvic floor reconstruction. I put up with symptoms for years without seeking further advice."

"If a man has ED he gets medical treatment, but addressing vaginal issues for women is seen as cosmetic 'rejuvenation'."

"That you can just have an operation and be fixed and go back to running, lifting, doing everything people saw you doing before."

"That it only affects women of a certain age."

"That having surgery to fix a uterus that falls out is considered an 'elective procedure'."

"That prolapse is not common, probably in part because no one (not even OB/GYNs) talk about it."

"That POP can only be repaired using mesh."

"That you're going to need a hysterectomy eventually."

"It's all in your head."

"You couldn't possibly have a prolapse because you have never birthed a child."

"That most physicians understand prolapse when they clearly don't. They misdiagnose all the time."

"That it's rare."

"Bottom of Form That my degree of prolapse didn't 'match my symptoms'. Like I'm just not trying hard enough or something."

"Prolapse is normal and there's not much you can do to help it or prevent it."

"That having a C-section or not having a baby prevents POP."

"I had to forcefully insist that my OBGYN check me for POP because 'it only happens to old women'. He checked me only on my insistence, then said 'wow that'll need surgery'. I was 28."

"That women would know if they had it. They'll be dealing with symptoms for years but since their doctor never mentioned it and nothing is yet visible outside, they assume it can't be prolapse."

"Kegels always help." Women may start doing Kegels by themselves at home for self-care and not realize you can do them wrong or that it will make a hypertonic floor worse."

"That it's perfectly fine to carry your heavy toddler despite research indicating heavy lifting causes POP."

"My Dr said to me, 'millions of women have rectocele, and they don't have pain'. Made me feel weak, worthless, and as though this is in my head. It isn't in my head."

"That urine leakage is normal like they portray in incontinence pad commercials."

"That having POP means you won't be able to live an active life or

exercise anymore."

"Assumption that with POP, the pelvic floor is weak. Not always the case."

"Many women can't use a pessary'. Well, more women would be able to use a pessary if they were offered different types and proper guidance."

"That women just know this stuff. It's a secret even in the medical community!!"

"That a hernia in your abdominal or groin area should be addressed right away, but a hernia in colon is no big deal."

"That you can't have sex if you have a prolapse."

Clearly, patient voice shines a light on POP reality.

"Sherrie Palm has compiled a comprehensive resource for patients with pelvic floor disorders, written using terms that patients can easily understand and admixed with real-life patient experiences. This book provides valuable information and destigmatizes common vulvovaginal conditions."

Cheryl Iglesia, MD

Women certainly don't join the POP community voluntarily. Once in the club, their membership often lasts a lifetime. Despite treatments, the body continues to age, and pelvic floor changes may continue to manifest because every woman has a unique lifestyle, behaviors, and co-existing conditions. Self-educating and self-awareness are key to moving forward.

NEXT STEPS

22

HEALTHCARE TUNNEL VISION

APOPS Patient Perspective: *"Finding APOPS was like finding an oasis when you are dying of thirst. There were thousands of other women in their space who understood everything I was experiencing, and their voices lifted me up through some of the very darkest nights of my journey."*

~SR, Germany

The problem with tunnel vision is we lose sight of valuable perceptions outside of the tunnel. Patient voice plays an integral role in the advancement of clinical practice.

I engage in conversations every chance I get regarding pelvic organ prolapse. Opportunities to discuss a health topic that has been shrouded in secrecy for thousands of years provide a gateway to healthcare evolution. As an advocate who guides women toward medical professionals for both surgical and nonsurgical treatment of POP, I encourage full disclosure of symptoms and concerns that are often embarrassing to discuss. I feel strongly that we need to get past the discomfort zone and recognize that at its most basic level, pelvic organ prolapse is a health condition that is treatable, not a subject that needs to be stuffed behind closed doors.

POP is a common, cryptic health concern considered "not that big of a deal" by some members of the medical community, possibly because it is not life-threatening like cancer or heart disease. But POP is a big deal, creating diverse QOL issues for an estimated 1 in 2 women from mid-teens through end-of-life. When we factor in the global scale of POP prevalence and the nearly 4,000 years of impact to women's quality of life, it is clear medical systems need to tune in. POP disables women from participating in typical activities, reducing and often eliminating the capacity to engage, causes physical discomfort and emotional difficulties, impacts employment, decreases fitness engagement, engenders social isolation, causes sexual dysfunction, and depletes self-esteem. POP often leads to exploration of multiple types of nonsurgical treatments and at times multiple surgical procedures because of the shortfall in diagnostic clinician curriculum, insufficient screening, and delayed referral to women's pelvic health specialists.

Women need to know that they are not alone, that millions of other women are experiencing the same frustrations at any given point in time. I am hopeful that in the near future women's wellness POP protocol will optimize pelvic floor health screenings and diagnostics ahead of the curve rather than after the fact. We have a long journey ahead of us.

Clinicians obviously must base treatment on curriculum and actionable experiences occurring throughout medical school, internship, residency, and fellowship. Unfortunately, emphasis placed on listening to patient feedback throughout the process is often insufficient in the process. Women with pelvic organ prolapse simply want their clinicians to listen to them. To believe them. To treat them with the same respect we give our healthcare providers even if what we are disclosing to them flies in the face of what their medical training has taught them about pelvic organ prolapse.

POP is a very diverse condition. The POP lesson to practitioners is pretty simple. Believe patients who share that they are experiencing pain or discomfort whether prior to treatment or after. Recognize that loss of intimacy is incredibly frustrating, and that POP invades the normalcy of patients' lives in a substantial way. Self-esteem takes a beating when experiencing POP.

The message to women is also pretty simple. Hold your heads high, disclose your symptoms in entirety, and insist on your healthcare professional spending the time due you to discuss your treatment options. It is vital to recognize that at their core, healthcare professionals are human, have good days and bad just like patients, are incredibly busy treating a multitude of patients and sometimes unintentionally get stuck in tunnel vision, treating all patients with pelvic organ prolapse the same, when needs are incredibly unique from woman to woman.

Every generation of women since the dawn of the civilized world has engaged to some degree in the momentum of women's health awareness and empowerment directives. In communications with those I've met along my journey to increase awareness of pelvic organ prolapse, I've heard countless stories regarding the QOL impacts to women's lives. Fortunately, the world at large is finally coming to terms with the reality of POP, and as women's voices become stronger and louder, the stigma that shrouds POP in silence will dissipate.

The big picture is as simple as it is for any other stigmatized health concern. There was a time no one could say the word breast out loud; we now freely and proudly shout our support of breast health campaigns and encourage open dialogue. The time has finally arrived to open the closet door and eradicate the stigma of pelvic organ prolapse. POP is a health condition, nothing more, nothing less.

As we enlighten the world at large regarding POP reality, we enable women to comfortably share stories about their very personal journeys. As we become more open-minded about what is without a doubt one of the most prevalent medical conditions women collectively experience, stigma will soften. Like most health concerns, awareness and open dialogue walk hand in hand to establish the new normal.

Given that childbirth and menopause are the leading causes of POP, this condition has and will continue to exist as long as women inhabit this planet. Regardless the geographic, ethnic, socio-economic, sociocultural, or theological backdrop, nearly all women will have at least one risk factor for experiencing POP because most women who live long enough will experience menopause. It is unfortunate that many women currently choose to live out their lives in physical discomfort because they either don't understand what is occurring in their bodies or they are too embarrassed to talk about it.

"Medical care has become corporatized in the late 20th and 21st centuries. Your personal physician is an employee, no longer your personal 'ombudsman' in the healthcare system. Added to this is physicians' historical disinterest in interacting directly and helpfully with sexual matters. Engage your practitioner with notes and with questions; be specific regarding the pros and cons of each therapeutic option, and do not leave without clarifying and getting answers to your sexual and aesthetic concerns. Ask your surgeon to repeat what she/he feels you have said. If you do not lobby for yourself, no one will do it for you."

Michael Goodman, MD

Above and beyond the quality-of-life impact of POP is the basic need to feel healthy. When a woman must spend day after day with considerable POP impact to daily activities, it is difficult to functionally focus on anything else. As women, we are not trying to recapture the bodies we had at the age of 25. Superficial aspects of childbirth like stretch marks don't rattle our cages; that is a fair price to pay for the miracle of motherhood. We accept the shift in our shapes that comes after bearing children. At the end of the day, what women with POP want is to simply feel normal again.

Ultimately, it is up to each woman as an individual to find the path that best addresses her quest to address POP symptoms. For some it may be as simple as a pessary for support, for some it may be a combination of nonsurgical treatments; and for some it may be surgical repair. It is essential women find a qualified clinician that fits their unique needs and move forward.

And it is imperative women with POP share what they learn along their journey and continue to push POP awareness forward to enable future generations of women to live in a world that recognizes, acknowledges, understands, and effectively addresses the extremely intricate and intimate impact of pelvic organ prolapse to our lives. Without a doubt, POP will engender the next significant evolution of and revolution in women's health.

23

THE ART OF ACCEPTANCE: A PIVOTAL STEP IN PELVIC ORGAN PROLAPSE HEALING

APOPS Patient Perspective: *"I really think if it wasn't for APOPS, I wouldn't make it. I have been struggling with this for eight years. What we experience and what doctors learn in school are two entirely different things. Without the knowledge and support I've gained from this group I would be lost.*

~ST, Israel

We are different; we are the same. While every woman must travel her own unique pelvic organ prolapse journey, the range of emotions we go through individually is as distinct as the color of our eyes. At some point in time, most POP sisters experience a relatively similar ride through that range of emotions. The most difficult emotion to balance regarding pelvic organ prolapse is *acceptance.*

PELVIC ORGAN PROLAPSE is the BIGGEST SECRET IN WOMEN'S HEALTH

Patient Voice Clarifies how POP Makes Women Feel

Defective, frustrated, isolated, stunned, alone, shocked, broken, embarrassed, weird, handicapped, sloppy, damaged, freaky, limited, imprisoned, uncomfortable, disgusting, empty, violated, disabled, fearful, vacant, wasted, lonely, gross, weak, droopy, destroyed, limited, ruined, depressed, solitary, hopeless, scared, old, ashamed, pained, worried, drained, misguided, betrayed, forsaken, angry, defeated, cheated, demoralized, deformed, suicidal, useless, failure, robbed, gross, grieving, afraid, cautious, nervous, vulnerable, limited, devastated, weird, forlorn, abnormal, helpless, silenced, guarded, invisible, terrified, hindered, unlovable, broken, repulsive, ashamed, hurting, imprisoned, marginalized, unfeminine.

Pelvic organ prolapse self esteem impact. Image courtesy of Association for Pelvic Organ Prolapse Support.

Women make themselves crazy with an endless list of questions. How did POP happen? Why is POP happening to me? Did I do something to cause POP? Why wasn't I warned about POP ahead of the curve? What should I do to fix my POP? Will my POP ever be cured? Can others tell I have POP? The destructive self-doubt keeps women up at night and haunts their days, especially immediately following diagnosis, because most women have no awareness of the condition prior to that point.

It is imperative we "see" ourselves. I'm not talking get the mirror out and look at your vagina (although that is a good preliminary self-diagnostic tool for women early in the learning curve). I don't mean analyze what degree of POP impact you are experiencing on any given day. I'm talking about look deep inside; what do we really need to be happy, to be whole? Is having a perfect body a necessity? Not even close.

> *"Self-acceptance is acknowledging one's flaws and virtues, physically and emotionally, without self-judgment or blame."*
>
> Hichem Bensmail, MD

When going through the bazillion emotions women experience when diagnosed with POP, it is helpful to share anxiety and fear but also hope with other women experiencing this extremely common but rarely openly acknowledged female health condition. Women newly diagnosed, women prepping for surgery, women in the post-surgical heal curve, women who have no interest in surgery all have anxiety and doubts. It is part of the learning curve, figuring out what tools work best for each of our unique bodies. The bravery of letting ourselves be seen and connecting with other women experiencing POP shores up our vulnerability.

Positive emotions influence the way we feel as well as the way we think. Are women upset to be diagnosed with a condition that has considerable physical, emotional, social, sexual, fitness, and employment quality of life impact? Absolutely. Should we allow ourselves to experience all emotions? Without a doubt. But should we let POP define us? Never.

Pelvic organ prolapse is a bump in the road - certainly a significant bump, but one that can be overcome with the strength and determination that defines most women today. We must recognize and celebrate everything bright and beautiful about ourselves with the simplicity we embrace as young children. Acceptance leads to healing.

A LEAP OF HOPE

24

My POP Experience

APOPS Patient Perspective: "*I discovered APOPS by accident. As a 40-something woman, not even being aware of pelvic organ prolapse tells you everything about the stigma, extreme lack of focus, education, and awareness surrounding this major health issue for women. Thank goodness this landscape is now changing, empowering women to lobby for change!*"

~SS, UK

I had a hysterectomy on my 40th birthday. Several large fibroids, a cyst-covered ovary, and aggressive adenomyosis (benign growth of tissue that embeds into the uterus) were making day-to-day function painful and frustrating. Despite an abdominal incision, I felt better 2 weeks' post-hysterectomy than I'd felt the entire year prior. To say I was delighted to have my uterus and one ovary removed is a bit of an understatement.

I had asked my gynecologist prior to my hysterectomy "what stops stuff from falling out?" I pictured the top end of the vaginal canal open and organs or tissues "dropping down the hole". As it turned out, tissues pushing down the vaginal canal was an actual concern. It would have been great if after I had opened the door to prolapse concerns with my gynecologist (albeit blindly), she would have taken the initiative to have a conversation explaining potential POP concerns. In retrospect, knowing what I know now, I can't blame my doctor.

I experienced POP symptoms prior to my hysterectomy. Difficulty keeping a tampon in. Years of chronic constipation. Vaginal pressure. I did not mention these issues to my gynecologist prior to my hysterectomy; perhaps if I had, our conversation would have gone in a different direction. It is important to ask the right questions and share all symptoms when discussing pelvic health with your physician.

> *"The Silent Epidemic. Pelvic Organ Prolapse. Many gynecologists run away from this and ignore the problems. Urologists don't want to deal with rectums falling out. They had to build a whole new subspecialty to focus on the problem. Yet, the general public still lives in darkness. I have seen this in my 30+ year career as a urogynecologist. So now I have a friend that brings light to this issue of POP and is a champion for women worldwide. Without her advocate role many women would continue to suffer in silence physically and emotionally. Sherrie's goal in her professional life is to educate and bring to the front the hope of relief, the hope of care, the hope of cure. We need Sherrie to teach us and help us understand how to address women's needs to hold back this Silent Epidemic."*
>
> Red Alinsod, MD

The next POP symptom my body displayed about 13 years later was difficulty starting my urine stream. I experienced this symptom for a notable amount of time but didn't question it. I would wake up in the middle of the night with an urge to urinate and would become frustrated because it was such a struggle to release the urine. I would massage my abdomen, listen to water running from the faucet, I even tried closing my eyes and visualizing a man urinating off a waterfall, to no avail. I would then return to massaging my abdomen, which would eventually enable the urine to flow. I now know that my urethra was crimped from POP displacement of organs and tissues, a common occurrence in advanced grades of POP severity. Abdominal massage managed to move and uncrimp the urethra, "opening up the hose" so to speak.

The POP symptom that finally got my attention was the tissue bulging out of my vagina. After feeling that lump for a few months, I finally became curious enough to get a hand-held mirror and took a look. I highly recommend women visually explore their vulva and vagina whether they suspect POP or not. This intimate zone of women's bodies is hidden from sight and is as unique from woman to woman as our faces. If viewing a lump coming out of your vagina isn't enough to convince you to get to a doctor, I don't know what is. In my case, the view was a walnut-sized lump bulging out of my vaginal canal. I had no idea what it was, all

I knew was that it wasn't normal, and I wanted it fixed.

I went to see my physician, who is also a close friend, and a pelvic exam was the next step. Upon examining me, she calmly advised me I had pelvic organ prolapse, that she would fit me with a pessary, and that if I wasn't happy with the pessary, she would refer me to a good urogynecologist for surgical evaluation. I had no clue what any of those terms meant. I'd never heard of POP prior to my diagnosis. That was the beginning of a momentous shift in my life, both physically and professionally. My physician fitted me with a pessary, and I was very fortunate that she identified the correct type and fit on her first attempt, relatively uncommon with pessary fitting.

The pessary worked well. Like contact lens for eyes fitted properly, once inserted you barely feel a pessary inside the vaginal canal. Despite a couple frustrating days getting used to inserting and removing my pessary (which included comical chase scenes when my pessary sprung out of my hand), I adapted pretty quickly to inserting the pessary in the morning and removing it at night to allow my tissues to breath and move freely with nothing rubbing on them. However, I quickly became frustrated with the need to insert and remove the pessary daily because of my extensive work schedule, so my doctor referred me to the top urogynecologist that she knew.

I'm not one to beat around the bush when it comes to self-educating regarding matters of my health. I did my homework, embedding myself in the internet as I hovered for my appointment. I went to see the urogynecologist armed with a sheet full of questions. After she completed a thorough pelvic and rectal exam, she advised me I had 2 of the 5 types of POP. She patiently took her time addressing every question I had. We then discussed the if and when of surgical repair. It was obvious that I had POP issues that needed to be addressed (my rectocele and cystocele were grade 3 and a large enterocele was additionally discovered during surgery). I wanted the surgery immediately. We booked surgery a month out. I took advantage of that time to continue my POP research in order to build a book to share the information I captured with other women. I knew if I wasn't familiar with pelvic organ prolapse after being so proactive with my health, other women likely weren't aware of it either.

I was exasperated that I needed surgery to fix something that was quite common but that I'd never heard of or read about. I questioned my surgeon how on earth that could be; she looked me right in the eye and stated matter-of-factly "Sherrie, women won't talk about POP". I was shocked and furious. I could not believe women would not talk about POP when they freely share the gory details of childbirth. My urogynecologist shared a story about how she had tried to bring the subject up at a book club, a group full of educated women, and it still did not get discussed. She said it is something that women just don't feel comfortable talking about.

From my initial diagnosis forward, I felt that this is a subject that *all* women need to know about. We live in an enlightened society. We are repetitively bombarded with every physical, emotional, social, and sexual tidbit of health information on television and the radio, as well as in books and magazines. Why not POP? I started to discuss POP with other women, and it was clear that I was not the only person in the dark.

Once I made the decision to have surgery, it was full speed ahead as far as I was concerned. I've never been one to ignore a health concern, whether for a health issue that needed surgery or a bandage. I feel it is critical women who want surgery to repair POP explore it from the most positive angle - get examined, repaired, heal, get on with your life. Dwelling in anxiety on the negative side of having POP or needing surgery to repair it has no benefit.

Like many women experiencing POP, I had multiple risk factors and will never know for certain what caused my POP issues, but I can make a pretty good guess.

Childbirth is validated as the leading causal factor, and I had one complication-free vaginal birth at the age of 35.

My mother had cystocele and rectocele issues, so there was a genetic factor.

I was diagnosed with MS at the age of 30, and despite a very negative wheelchair-bound prognosis when it was initially identified, I have kept MS under control over the years since then. But women with neuromuscular disorders are predisposed to POP because of loss of muscle strength. Additionally, those who are wheelchair-bound are susceptible to atrophied muscle tissue.

Although I've not regretted my hysterectomy for a second, hysterectomy is a documented POP causal concern since the removal of a large organ in the center of pelvic organs can clearly cause organ or tissue shift. Years of chronic constipation from stress-related IBS was another factor.

Zero doubt decrease in muscle tissue strength and integrity from menopausal estrogen loss compounded my risk.

I spent a few summers landscaping my yard with considerable heavy lifting that included moving large boulders and shoveling multiple yards of gravel, undoubtedly detrimental to my pelvic floor.

Like most women with POP, I had multiple risk factors and will never know the cause definitively, but at the post-repair point, my main concern is and will always be adjusting lifestyle and behaviors that are known to be damaging to the pelvic floor.

Notably, over the years prior to my POP diagnosis I recognized a loss of PC muscle strength. I have always had strong awareness of my pelvic floor. The fact that I noticed I was having a harder time contracting this muscle, even though I really did not experience much of a problem with urine leakage unless I was jumping up and down and screaming while watching football, indicates that I had been cognizant of my body's red flags.

Maintenance for life means assessing lifestyle and behaviors and avoiding those that generate risk whether mesh is used for surgical POP repair or not. The pelvic floor and core exercise regimen included in my daily maintenance routine help maintain strength in critical muscle structures. I've experimented over the years with multiple core and pelvic floor strengthening regimens and devices. I continue to review new programs and include a mixture of exercises from different programs within my regimen. It is essential women utilize a program that best fits their individual needs. We are all unique and what works for one may not necessarily be appropriate for another.

I'd like to pass along a few personal notes about my post-surgical period, and it is important to recognize that everyone's surgical experience is different. Our body types, the kinds of POP being repaired, the degree of severity we experience, our lifestyles, our behaviors, even our co-existing health conditions impact surgical outcomes. I was very uncomfortable that first week after surgery and by and large lived on the couch. However, I did go off narcotic pain medication on the third day post-surgery because I react strongly to nearly all of them. By the second week, I was up and moving around freely. I noticed the swelling and discomfort became more pronounced which of course was because I was upright and moving. By the end of the second week, I was walking relatively normally; by week three the bruising was gone (expect a lot of bruising, as in a completely black and blue crotch). At 3 weeks, I continued to use the beanbag heat pad for pain control while I watched TV at night. At this point, I could comfortably wear jeans.

Several months post-surgery, I noticed a pressure sensation while exercising. I requested an appointment with my surgeon and after a thorough checkup, she assured me everything was fine. Since I am fairly hands-on with weight training (free weights, ten-pound maximum), my surgeon recommended that when I lift anything heavy over the next few months, I insert a tampon to contain downward pressure. I questioned whether I should use a pessary for this purpose, and she said that there should be no need to. Mesh was used to repair both my cystocele and rectocele; this was a protective measure to prevent POP recurrence considering I am extremely active. I used the tampon support method while weight training for 1 month and after that, my tissues were strong enough to handle lifting two 10-pound dumbbells. I continue to evaluate whether items I lift are too heavy however, to maintain my repair long term.

On the sexual activity front, once I got past the initial post-surgical heal curve, I slowly resumed intimacy with no problems. Note, do not engage in intimacy until your surgeon releases you to do so or you may damage repairs. As a woman who enjoys her sexuality, it was extremely important to me to be able to engage in an active sex life as well as enjoy it. The core location of sexual sensation shifted, and the sensations seemed more intense. I'm not sure if this is because the pressure that the prolapsed organs put on the nerves in the area prevented sensation or if there was no discomfort to distract from the pleasure sensations. Initially I was unable to orgasm, and over time that shifted to being fully orgasmic again. Nerves take longer to heal than any other tissue; be patient.

Since every woman's POP surgical experience will be unique, it's best to have some idea in mind of what is to come. The more questions you ask prior to a POP procedure, the less anxiety you will experience. There is zero doubt in my mind that POP surgery was a smart choice for me. At three months, I felt fairly healed up with minor pain at a couple of the laparoscopic incision sites. (I had 6 laparoscopic incisions plus vaginal incisions). It took six months to a year before I completely felt like I had prior to my POP procedure. Do not expect to be 100% back to normal within the 6-8 week heal curve most surgeons suggest. If I had to make the choice all over again whether to have surgery to repair pelvic organ prolapse, I wouldn't hesitate for a moment to have surgery for POP repair.

25

THE EVOLUTION OF WOMEN'S PELVIC EXAMS: POP SCREENING, DIAGNOSTICS, AND TREATMENT

APOPS Patient Perspective: *"My doctor smiled and mentioned that I was the smartest patient he ever had. I have APOPS and Sherrie Palm to thank for that!"*

~SR, Illinois/USA

Like most women, I had never heard of pelvic organ prolapse, a urogynecologist, or a pessary. Next step for me was doing what everyone else on the planet would do, hit Dr. Google. And the more information I found, the angrier I got. When I was diagnosed in 2007, 3.3 million women in the US were estimated to experience POP. I can't begin to imagine how unsettling it is for women who are newly diagnosed today and discover that 50% of women is currently a common POP prevalence estimate in studies.

In the years that have passed since the destiny diverting day I stepped into the pelvic organ prolapse advocacy arena, much has shifted. There's good news and bad on the POP front lines. Despite the difficulties navigating the transvaginal mesh mess that exploded in the United States in 2011, the end result was beneficial. The majority of POP surgeries are now performed by subspecializing fellowship trained urogynecologists and urologists. Medical devices are continually evolving and are researched and regulated more strictly. Innovative nonsurgical treatments are continually coming to the forefront. Treatment options for women continue to expand and advance.

However, while the treatment side of POP moves forward, little has shifted regarding inclusion of POP in women's pelvic wellness screening protocol. Little has shifted regarding development of POP curriculum to appropriately educate diagnostic clinicians about the why, when, and how to appropriately screen for POP. And little has shifted in POP awareness and open dialogue during women's wellness exams.

> *"Finding the best provider is key when it comes to dealing with POP, whether minimally invasive solutions or surgical options for managing your condition."*
>
> Debra Muth, ND

POP was not openly discussed during pelvic wellness exams back in 2007 when I was diagnosed. It is still not openly discussed today during women's wellness screenings. A common question women newly diagnosed with POP ask is *why wasn't I informed of or screened for pelvic organ prolapse sooner?* Research abstracts and articles are available online, but clinician/patient discussions rarely wander into the POP zone unless women initiate the conversation regarding symptoms they are experiencing. And if they are too embarrassed to ask the right questions, the POP screening may not occur at all.

When I was diagnosed with POP, I wanted to shout it to the world in a fit of rage. I was furious that despite the pandemic prevalence of this common, diverse condition, I was given no forewarning. It did not make sense to me then. It does not make sense to me now. Childbirth and menopause are the leading POP causal factors. Women's wellness screening includes a routine pelvic exam, but POP exploration is not standard practice during pelvic exams, despite pandemic prevalence and very widespread causal factors. What's wrong with this picture?

As in every underrecognized aspect of health, we don't know what we don't know. Every single woman newly diagnosed with or suspecting she has POP because she's googled her symptoms online, must travel a diverse path of self-discovery. Five types of POP, four grades of severity, numerous types of POP occurring simultaneously, diverse symptoms that may or may not occur, multiple nonsurgical treatment choices, an abundance of surgical options, difference of opinion among healthcare professionals - the list of variables goes on and on. The only universal denominator with POP is the fact that it occurs in women.

- infertility 10%
- bacterial vaginosis 29%
- yeast infections 75%
- UTI 40%
- abnormal uterine bleeding 9-14%
- fibroids 70%, surgery 30%
- ovarian cysts 18%
- polycystic ovary syndrome 15%
- rectal bleeding 9-11%
- endometriosis 2-10%
- tumors of genital tissues 1-2%
- genital warts 10%
- STD's 20%
- POP 50%-no screening?

VAGINAL HEALTH

PELVIC EXAM includes the vagina, cervix, uterus, ovaries, rectum

Pelvic exam standards of practice. Image courtesy of Association for Pelvic Organ Prolapse Support.

Every time I communicate with women struggling to dissect the maze, I feel the steps to stimulate open POP discussion are taking too long. If our gynecologists, primary care physicians, midwives, and other healthcare practitioners who provide pelvic exams aren't educated on the prevalence of POP and the need for routine screening, how is the status quo ever going to improve? We need to talk about pelvic organ prolapse. We need to talk about pelvic organ prolapse OUT LOUD. Silence should no more encase vaginal and pelvic health than any other aspect of women's wellness.

Not a day goes by that I don't wander upon an intriguing new POP insight, statistic, article, study, or conversation shining unique light on the diverse layers of pelvic organ prolapse. To say my world is buried in layers of information I wish I could absorb by osmosis is an understatement. But the POP silence in healthcare is staggering. While we certainly should celebrate the many advances and changing societal perceptions in women's health that have occurred in previous generations, it is imperative we remain both cognizant and at times critical of stagnation within the POP space. There is little doubt it's time to advance pelvic organ prolapse directives into the 21st century.

26

WOMEN'S HEALTH EMPOWERMENT: THE FINAL FRONTIER

APOPS Patient Perspective: *"As a 40 something woman, not even being aware of pelvic organ prolapse tells you everything about the stigma, extreme lack of focus, education, and awareness surrounding this major health issue for women. Thank goodness APOPS is now changing the landscape, empowering women to lobby for change."*
~SS, Utah/USA

A lthough progress has occurred regarding comprehensive and coordinated women's healthcare, a significant practice gap remains.

As women, our collective health depends on our willingness to talk openly and comfortably about vaginal health with our healthcare practitioners, but also among ourselves as a female culture. The evolution of women's communal health rests heavily on what we are comfortable sharing with our mothers, daughters, sisters, friends, and of course our intimate partners. Social acceptance is a marker of women's health empowerment. Somehow pelvic organ prolapse (POP) remains a pariah in women's wellness.

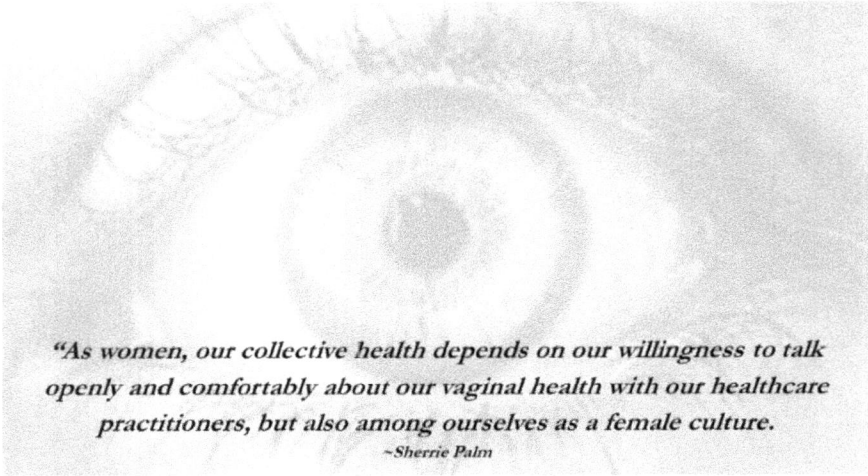

"As women, our collective health depends on our willingness to talk openly and comfortably about our vaginal health with our healthcare practitioners, but also among ourselves as a female culture."
~Sherrie Palm

Multiple conditions throughout the history of women's health have had to over-come the stigma of sexual connotation to enable open public dialogue, such as breast health and reproductive rights. The biggest barrier we have yet to conquer is related to vaginal health in general and most often, pelvic organ prolapse specific. While medically documented dating back to 1835 B.C., we have yet to break down the POP wall of silence. Women are seldom informed of POP ahead of the curve. Discovery upon diagnosis runs rampant regarding this common, cryptic women's health pandemic.

> *"Vaginal childbirth has been destroying vaginas since the beginning of time and modern pelvic floor research has been confirming what mothers have known for generations."*
>
> Marco Pelosi III, MD

We live in a society that worships comparative perfection. While the opinions of others are irrelevant in the big picture, self-image is a significant marker of self-confidence. The plethora of hair, face, and body cosmetic items available clarifies our need for body perfection, and marketing campaigns are skilled at encouraging artful deception on the outside. How we really feel about how we look digs a bit deeper. The reality is women all too often suffer in silence with vaginal health issues that impact self-image yet remain hidden behind a wall of silence.

Shouldn't we talk about ALL women's health concerns out loud? Form, feel, function and personal perception of the vagina and vulva are critical for optimization of vaginal and intimate health sense of self. Behind blissful birthing stories exists a cryptic aftermath that seldom makes it into the public forum. Tissues bulging out of the vagina, wide vaginal gap, coital incontinence, and pain with intimacy are very common after-effects of vaginal childbirth and very real to the women experiencing them. At times, horrific birthing experiences result in ravaged vaginal, rectal, and perineal tissue that leave women with pain and dysfunction for years, sometimes the rest of their lives, because they don't know where to go to address the problem.

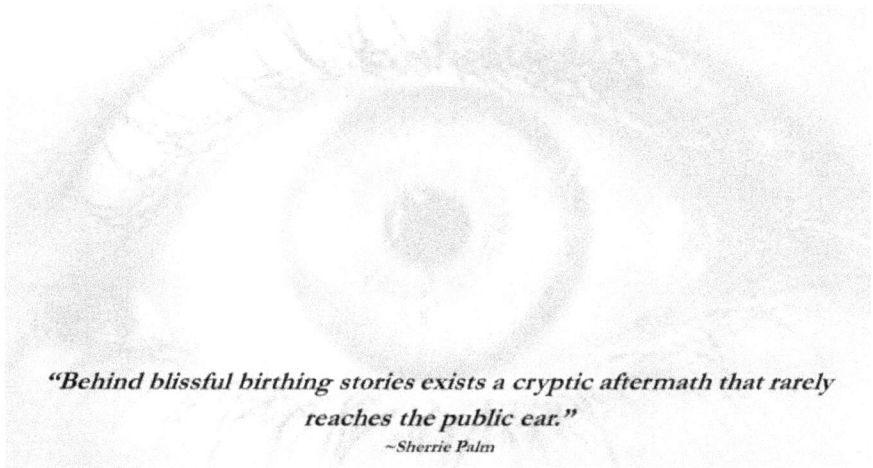

"Behind blissful birthing stories exists a cryptic aftermath that rarely reaches the public ear."
~Sherrie Palm

Although progress has occurred regarding comprehensive and coordinated women's wellness screening, a significant awareness gap still exists regarding vaginal health. What is the secret sauce to destigmatize and enable all women to talk out loud comfortably about the QOL impacts of pelvic organ prolapse? The complexity of pelvic organ prolapse necessitates a comprehensive approach to evolve women's wellness screening, along with a multidisciplinary approach to springboard early detection and treatment.

During the breast cancer awareness transition in the 20th century prior to which breast health remained a highly stigmatized, unspoken health issue, women in positions of celebrity or political power stepped forward, associating themselves with breast health concerns. Because a few brave women with influence were willing to share their stories, breast health awareness advanced and eradicated the obscuring stigma of what had been previously viewed as off-the-table erogenous dialogue.

The courageous efforts of Terese Lasser, Founder of Reach to Recovery.

Seventeen magazine editor Babette Rosmond, author of *The Invisible Worm*, challenging assumptions of surgeons treating women with breast cancer.

Actress Shirley Temple Black sharing her story in McCall's magazine.

Former First Lady Betty Ford and Happy Rockefeller, wife of Vice-President Nelson Rockefeller, sharing their diagnoses via televised press conferences.

NBC news correspondent Betty Rollin writing *First You Cry* about her experiences.

Each of these brave women increased media exposure and engendered a new era in women's breast health empowerment. We need highly prominent women in positions of visibility and voice to do the same regarding pelvic organ prolapse, ushering in the next significant revolution in women's health empowerment.

We must disrupt women's healthcare due process. While we certainly should celebrate the many advances and changing societal perceptions in women's health that have occurred in prior generations, it is imperative we remain cognizant and at times critical of stagnation.

Healthcare should include delivery models shaped by female experience. But if women are not talking out loud about these experiences, and healthcare does not recognize or acknowledge the pandemic needs, how do we break down the barriers? Gaps in medical curriculum create roadblocks to delivery of much-needed services. FemTech dialogue looms large these days, typically addressing fertility, menstruation, menopause, and sexual health but rarely acknowledging the POP pandemic.

Healthcare should be accessible, preventative, proactive, and evidence-based. Evolving care models create potential to overcome the current shortfall in the remaining stigmatized vaginal healthcare zone. It is imperative we ensure that medical disciplines of all specialties addressing basic women's wellness are prepared to provide appropriate screening for POP to address needs as women flow through life transitions.

When women's shrouded health conditions are of pandemic prevalence, as is the case for POP, we must make every effort to tear down the last walls of stigmatized silence preventing access to care. The individual threads of the fabric of women's health policy must remain strong but flexible and forward-thinking.

When will we reach the comfort zone with pelvic organ prolapse? Until the world at large effectively talks out loud about this common women's health issue, little forward momentum in vaginal health empowerment will occur.

Policymakers, clinical leaders, visionary entrepreneurs, and investors each have a role to play to close gaps and overcome barriers in vaginal and intimate wellness which remain highly stigmatized. Patient voice has a significant role to play as well; it must be encouraged by all sectors to break down barriers and fuel the revolution in vaginal health.

The power of community will override the silence. The resilience of women talking out loud about vaginal health will bring it to the forefront as it did breast health. Advocates, health systems, governments, and most of all women, must publicly acknowledge stigmatized women's health conditions to affect change.

When we ignore the nearly 4000 years of medical documentation of pelvic organ prolapse, we dismiss women's health empowerment.

When we talk about incontinence jokingly and simply slap a pad on it as though it is not a big deal, we dismiss women's health empowerment.

When we block efforts to talk out loud about vaginal and intimate health in a respectful way, we dismiss women's health empowerment.

And when we as women choose to not engage in the POP conversation out loud, we disparage the efforts of so many of our foresisters who worked incredibly hard for the evolution of women's wellness and best practice.

Every Voice Matters.

APPENDICES

APPENDIX A: TIPS AND TOOLS

TIPS

Bridging: Wash hands. Place the first two fingers against labia lips, apply gentle pressure to prevent a pessary from pushing out during defecation.

Splinting: Wash hands. Insert two fingers into the vagina and position them against the rear vaginal wall to push a rectocele bulge back into alignment to assist defecation.

Heavy lifting: Avoid whenever possible. Contract your pelvic floor prior to lifting a child or other heavy weight. Hold a child or other heavy weight close to the body if you must lift.

Trust your judgment, avoid activities that create pressure on the pelvic floor.

Avoid strain during bowel movements despite constipation.

If possible, sit while coughing to reduce pressure on your pelvic floor.

Cross your legs and bend at the waist prior to sneezing to reduce intra-abdominal pressure.

Request a standing pelvic exam when told POP is low-grade severity but you have pronounced POP symptoms.

Focus on what you can do, not on what you can't do, whether prior to or post-surgery.

Say no to work, family, friends regarding activities POP inappropriate.

Whether or not you choose to have POP surgery, optimize a life-long POP fitness regimen to maintain quality of life.

Seek guidance from a women's health physical therapist/physiotherapist prior to choosing a fitness activity, particularly if you have a hypertonic (tight) pelvic floor.

Core, pelvic floor, posture, and hip stability all play a role in pelvic organ prolapse maintenance. Kegels must be performed correctly to be effective, contracting the pelvic floor muscles up and in. Posture is important to reduce intra-abdominal pressure; pull your shoulders/chest up from your ribs with shoulders lifted up and pulled back. Contract your abdominal muscles, drawing your belly button up and in to support your core when possible.

Eat a diet high in produce fiber to avoid or reduce constipation.

Make your bowel and bladder happy, drink sufficient water.

Raise knees with feet resting on a stool while sitting on the toilet to ease defecation.

Lean forward with elbows resting on knees with feet flat on the floor to ease urination.

POST-SURGICAL TOOLS

- Ice bag

- Hydrocortisone 1% cream

- Colace Stool softener

- KY Jelly

- KY Ultra-Liquid or Liquid Silk

- Foam or inflatable donut seat cushion

- Baby sippee cup or cup with attached straw

- Sanitary napkins and panty-liners (no tampons)

- Baby wipes

- Loose clothing

- Pain medication

- Topical estrogen to aid healing of incisions if menopausal or peri-menopausal

CONSTIPATION TOOLS

- Magnesium

- MiraLAX

- Flaxseed

- Probiotics

- Water (increase intake)

- Sodium docusate stool softener

- Glycerin suppositories

- Squatty Potty or stool

FECAL INCONTINENCE AND FLATULENCE TOOLS

- Eclipse

- Butterfly Pads

- Imodium when traveling

- Gas-X

URINARY TRACT INFECTION TOOLS

- Cranberry supplement to help prevent a UTI

- Drink ample water to flush system

- AZO for discomfort

Appendix B: Resources

SUPPORT
Association for Pelvic Organ Prolapse Support (APOPS)

www.pelvicorganprolapsesupport.org

PHYSICIAN REVIEW SITES

www.ratemds.com

www.healthgrades.com

www.vitals.com

Google practitioners by name to explore Google ratings and review their websites. However, it is important to recognize that Google reviews do not always provide an accurate picture. Patients with successful outcomes often simply move on with their lives rather than post ratings. Patients with complications or physician/patient personality conflicts may post negative practitioner feedback.

APPENDIX C: POP RISK FACTOR QUESTIONNAIRE (POP-RFQ)

The POP-RFQ, available in 17 languages, can be downloaded from the APOPS website. Explore https://www.pelvicorganprolapsesupport.org/pop-risk-factor -questionnaire or Google APOPS + Risk Factor Questionnaire.

If you are experiencing pelvic, vaginal, or rectal symptoms and suspect you have pelvic organ prolapse, this questionnaire provides preliminary information to initiate POP screening by a healthcare clinician. If you answer yes to POP risk factors detailed on this questionnaire, request POP screening by a primary care physician or gynecologist. Circle the applicable answer on the printout.

1. Have you had at least one vaginal birth?
   Yes _____   No _____   Number of births? _____

2. Did you experience a long labor, forceps, or suction delivery?
   Yes _____   No _____

3. Do you see or feel tissues bulging from your vagina?
   Yes _____   No _____

4. Are you in menopause?
   Yes _____   No _____

5. Do you leak urine when you sneeze, cough, or laugh?
   Yes _____   No _____

6. Do you have difficulty starting your urine stream?
   Yes _____   No _____

7. Have you experienced stool leakage?
   Yes _____   No _____

8. Have you had chronic constipation for over a year?
   Yes _____   No _____

9. Do you lift heavy weights at home or work (including children over 30#)?
   Yes _____   No _____

10. Do you marathon run, jog, or engage in heavy-lifting athletic activities
    Yes _____   No _____

11. Have you had a hysterectomy?
    Yes _____   No _____

12. Do you experience chronic coughing from allergies or emphysema?
    Yes _____   No _____

13. Do your tampons push out of place
    Yes _____   No _____

14. Do you feel pelvic, back, rectal, or vaginal pain?
    Yes _____   No _____

15. Do you feel vaginal or rectal pressure?
    Yes _____   No _____

16. Is intercourse painful?
    Yes _____   No _____

17. Do you have reduced sexual sensation?
    Yes _____   No _____

18. Are you double-jointed or have really stretchy skin?
    Yes _____   No _____

This questionnaire is not meant to take the place of treatment from a health care practitioner. Always seek the advice of your physician on matters of personal health.

APPENDIX D: POP QUESTIONS TO ASK YOUR PHYSICIAN

A downloadable version of POP Questions To Ask Your Physician is available at https://www.pelvicorganprolapsesupport.org/pop-questions-to-ask-your-physician

1. What type(s) of POP do I have?

2. What grade of severity is my POP?

3. What are the nonsurgical treatment options?

4. What are the surgical treatment options?

5. What are the benefits and problems of using a pessary?

6. Will I be able to maintain my prolapse by doing pelvic floor exercises and using a pessary?

7. Will one surgery treat all of my different types of POP?

8. Will my surgery be vaginal, robotic, abdominal, or laparoscopic?

9. How many surgical incisions will I have?

10. Will mesh be used for my surgery?

11. What are my risks of mesh erosion?

12. How frequently do you provide this procedure, and what is your success

rate with it?

13. What are potential surgical complications?

14. How successful is this procedure at repairing POP long term?

15. If you find any problems with my uterus or ovaries during surgery, is there a chance they will be removed?

16. Will I need to stay in the hospital overnight after my procedure?

17. Will this procedure relieve all my symptoms? If not, which symptoms are likely to remain?

18. Will I need to be on narcotic pain medication after surgery and if so, for how long?

19. Will this surgery fix my urinary incontinence?

20. Will this surgery fix my fecal incontinence?

21. Will my constipation go away after surgery?

22. Will I need to wear a pessary after surgery?

23. How long will it take for sexual sensation to return?

24. How long will I need to wait to have sex after surgery?

25. Will this surgery impact my ability to have an orgasm?

26. Will sex be painful after my surgical repair has healed?

27. How long will I need to wait to return to my normal activities after surgery?

28. How long will I need to wait before I return to work after surgery?

29. How long should I wait to do pelvic floor maintenance exercises after surgery?

APPENDIX E: MESH QUESTIONS TO ASK YOUR PHYSICIAN

A downloadable version of Mesh Questions to Ask Your Physician is available at https://www.pelvicorganprolapsesupport.org/mesh

1. Do you plan to use mesh for my POP repairs?

2. How many mesh procedures like mine have you done?

3. What surgical alternatives do I have to mesh for repair?

4. Is there any reason I would be a bad candidate for mesh?

5. Will my POP repair be successful without mesh?

6. How long has the mesh product you use been on the market?

7. How long have you been using this particular mesh product?

8. Is there a chance mesh surgery won't fix my POP?

9. What side effects should I be concerned about after mesh surgery?

10. I am double-jointed and have really stretchy skin; will this increase risk of surgical mesh complications?

11. Will my partner be able to feel mesh during intimacy?

12. What are the chances mesh will erode with my surgery?

13. If I have mesh complications, will you be able to address them?

14. Can I have access to information on the mesh you will be using prior to having my surgical procedure?

APPENDIX F: ACRONYMS

A&P: Anterior/posterior pelvic organ prolapse repair

APOPS: Association for Pelvic Organ Prolapse Support

BHRT: Bioidentical hormone replacement therapy

CI: Coital incontinence

CUI: Coital urinary incontinence

DRA: Diastasis rectus abdominus

E1: Estrone

E2: Estradiol

E3: Estriol

EBD: Energy-based device

ED: Erectile dysfunction

EDS: Ehlers Danlos Syndrome

FDA: Food and Drug Administration

FI: Fecal Incontinence

FPMRS: Female pelvic medicine reconstructive surgeon

GERD: Gastroesophageal reflux disease

hEDS: Hypermobile Ehlers-Danlos syndrome

HIFEM: High-intensity focused electromagnetic wave technology

HRT: Hormone replacement therapy

IAP: Intra-abdominal pressure

IUD: Intrauterine device

LA: Levator avulsion

LAMi: Levator ani muscle injury

MFR: Myofascial release therapy

MUI: Mixed urinary incontinence

NIH: National Institutes of Health

OAB: Overactive bladder

OASIS: Obstetric anal sphincter injury

OTC: Over the counter

PAP: Pap smear

PC: Pubococcygeus muscle

POP: Pelvic organ prolapse

POP-Q: Pelvic organ prolapse quantification system

POP-RFQ: Pelvic organ prolapse risk factor questionnaire

PT: Physical therapy

PTNS: Posterior tibial nerve stimulation

QOL: Quality of life

RF: Radio frequency

RICE: Rest, ice, compression, and elevation,

SUI: Stress urinary incontinence

UI: Urinary incontinence

UTI: Urinary tract infection

UUI: Urge urinary incontinence

VTR: Vaginal tissue restoration or vaginal tissue regeneration

WHO: World Health Organization

GLOSSARY

adenomyosis: A benign inward growth of the uterine lining.

biofeedback: A technique for making bodily processes perceptible to the senses so that they can be controlled or manipulated.

bioidentical hormone replacement: Natural hormones manufactured from soybeans or wild yams which duplicate and replace the hormones whose levels fall during perimenopause and menopause.

bladder: The sac in the pelvic region that retains urine until it is excreted from the body.

bridging: Placement of the first two fingers against labia lips and applying gentle pressure to prevent a pessary from pushing out during defecation.

catheter: A flexible tube inserted into the bladder to drain urine.

coital incontinence: Involuntary loss of urine in association with sexual intercourse.

collagen: Fibrous protein in connective tissue.

colpocleisis: A POP surgical procedure to close off the vaginal opening.

cystocele: Prolapse in which the bladder shifts downward toward and into the vagina, pushing along with the front vaginal wall to the outside of the body.

cystoscopy: A medical test for viewing the bladder and urethra.

diastasis rectus abdominus: Separation of the left and right sides of the outermost abdominal (stomach) muscle.

defecography (proctography, dynamic rectal examination): A type of medical radiological imaging in which the mechanics of a patient's defecation are visualized in real-time using a fluoroscope.

elastin: A highly elastic protein in connective tissue that allows many tissues in the body to resume their shape after stretching or contracting.

enterocele: Prolapse in which the small intestine shifts down between the rectum and back wall of the vagina or between the uterus and front wall of the vagina.

estrogen: A group of hormones that generate female characteristics in the body.

Ehlers Danlos syndrome: A group of inherited disorders that affect your connective tissues — primarily your skin, joints, and blood vessel walls.

Female Pelvic Medicine Reconstructive Surgeon (FPMRS): A urogynecologist or urologist that specializes in clinical problems associated with dysfunction of the female pelvic floor, reproductive organs, bladder, and bowels.

fecal incontinence: The inability to control bowel movements, causing stool (feces) to leak unexpectedly from the rectum.

gastroesophageal reflux disease (GERD): Stomach acid repeatedly flows back into the tube connecting your mouth and stomach (esophagus)

hormone replacement therapy (HRT): Synthetic or natural hormone replacement to supplement depleted levels.

hysterectomy: Surgical removal of the uterus.

incontinence: Inability to retain urine within the bladder or feces within the colon.

intra-abdominal pressure: Steady state of pressure contained within the abdominal cavity.

irritable bowel: A chronic disorder of the colon characterized by alternating diarrhea and constipation.

Kegel exercises: Repetitive contractions of the pelvic floor pubococcygeus (PC) muscle that control the flow of urine and enhance sexual responsiveness.

labia: The external areas of female genital lip tissue surrounding the vagina and clitoris.

laparoscopic: Minimally invasive surgical procedure with small incisions.

levator ani: A broad, thin muscle situated on either side of the pelvis. It is formed from three muscle components: the puborectalis, the pubococcygeus muscle (which includes the puborectalis) and the iliococcygeus muscle and is attached to the inner surface of each side of the lesser pelvis, forming the greater part of the pelvic floor.

menopause: The natural regression of ovary function and cessation of menstruation.

mixed urinary incontinence: Mixture of both stress and urge urinary incontinence.

myofascial release therapy: A hands-on technique that involves applying gentle sustained pressure into the myofascial connective tissue restrictions to eliminate pain and restore motion.

obstetric anal sphincter injury (OASIS): Vaginal and perineal injuries complications that occur during vaginal delivery.

overactive bladder (OAB): Urinary urgency, with or without urgency-associated urinary incontinence.

pap smear: A screening test for cervical cancer named after Georgios Papanikolaou, MD.

PC muscle: The pubococcygeus muscle is a trampoline-like muscle that sits at the base of the pelvic cavity, supporting the organs and tissues of the pelvic region. This muscle is also responsible for the ability to start and stop the flow of urine and impacts level of sexual sensation in the vaginal area. Also referred to as the pelvic floor muscle.

pelvic exam: A routine gynecologic exam to check the internal and external tissues of the vagina, vulva, and labia.

pelvic floor muscles: Refer to PC muscle.

pelvic organ prolapse (POP): A condition in which an organ or organs and connecting tissues within the pelvic cavity shift in a downward direction out of their normal positions, toward or into the vaginal canal and surrounding area, and/or push outside of the body via the vagina.

peri-menopause: The period prior to menopause that is marked by fluctuating marked physical changes such as hot flashes or menstrual irregularity, due to a reduction of hormone levels.

pessary: A synthetic device inserted into the vagina to support pelvic organs and tissues.

POP: Pelvic organ prolapse, a female health condition in which an organ or organs and connecting tissues within the pelvic cavity shift in a downward direction out of their normal positions toward or into the vaginal canal and/or to the outside of the body.

POP-Q: Pelvic Organ Prolapse Quantification system provides characterization of a woman's prolapse and allows a uniform recording of degree of severity.

procidentia: The uterus pushes through the vaginal opening to rest completely outside of the body.

pubococcygeus muscle (PC): A trampoline-like muscle which sits at the base of the pelvic cavity, supporting organs and tissues above it, also referred to as the PC or pelvic floor muscle. This muscle is also responsible for the ability to start and stop the flow of urine and effects level of sexual sensation in the pubic/vaginal areas.

rectocele: Prolapse in which the rectum bulges into the rear vaginal wall.

speculum: Metal or plastic instrument used to hold the vagina open during a pelvic exam.

splinting: Inserting two fingers into the vagina and pushing against the vaginal wall to push a rectocele bulge back into alignment to enable defecation.

stress urinary incontinence (SUI): Urine leaks out with sudden pressure on the bladder and urethra, causing the sphincter muscles to open briefly.

tibial nerve stimulation: Neuromodulation therapy used to treat overactive bladder (OAB) and the associated symptoms of urinary urgency, urinary frequency, and urge incontinence.

urethra: The tube that carries urine away from the bladder to the outside of the body.

urethral bulking agents: A medical treatment used to treat urinary incontinence in women. Injectable materials are used to control stress incontinence.

uterine prolapse: Prolapse in which the uterus shifts down into the vagina and/or out of the body through the vaginal opening.

urinary incontinence: Inability to hold urine in the bladder due to loss of voluntary control over the urinary sphincters resulting in the involuntary passage of urine; stress urinary incontinence (SUI), urge urinary incontinence (UUI), and overactive bladder (OAB) are types of urinary incontinence.

uterus: Hollow, pear-shaped organ that is located in a woman's lower abdomen, between the bladder and the rectum in which babies develop prior to birth.

urge urinary incontinence: A strong urge to urinate with difficulty retaining urine until restroom access has occurred.

vagina: The muscular canal that extends between the uterus to the genital area outside of the body.

vaginal atrophy: An inflammation of the vagina (and the outer urinary tract) due to the thinning and shrinking of the tissues, as well as decreased lubrication.

vaginal vault prolapse: The top of the vagina caves in on itself after the uterus is removed (hysterectomy).

RESOURCES

Introduction

Forecasting the Prevalence of Pelvic Floor Disorders in U.S. Women: 2010 to 2050.

Jennifer Wu et al; 2009. Obstet Gynecol.

Chapter 1

Uterine Prolapse: From Antiquity to Today.

Keith T. Downing; 2012. Obstet Gynecol Int.

Prevalence of Pelvic Floor Disorders in Elderly Women: A Population-based Study.

Mathias A De Araújo et al; 2020. ICS2020 Online.

Surgical Updates in the Treatment of Pelvic Organ Prolapse.

Julia Geynisman-Tan et al; 2017. Rambam Maimonides Med J.

Cost of Pelvic Organ Prolapse Surgery in the United States.

Leslee L Subak et al; 2001. ResearchGate.

Chapter 3

Childbirth and Pelvic Floor Dysfunction: An Epidemiologic Approach to the Assessment of Prevention Opportunities at Delivery.

Divya A. Patel et al; 2006. Am J Obstet Gynecol.

Evidence for Pelvic Organ Prolapse Predisposition Genes on Chromosomes 10 and 17.

Kristina Allen-Brady et al; 2014. Am J Obstet Gynecol.

Hysterectomy.NWHN Staff; 2015. National Women's Health Network.

A Study of Bladder Dysfunction in Women with Type 2 Diabetes Mellitus.

Sanjay Bhat, et al; 2014. Indian J Endocrinol Metab.

The Prevalence of Urinary Incontinence among Adolescent Female Athletes: A Systematic Review.

Tamara Rial Rebullido, et al; 2021. J Funct Morphol Kinesiol.

Post-hysterectomy Vaginal Vault Prolapse.

Dudley Robinson, et al; 2018. ScienceDirect.

Chapter 4

Diagnosis and Comparative Effectiveness of Treatments for Urinary Incontinence in Adult Women.

AHRQ Staff, 2010. Agency for Healthcare Research and Policy

Female Urinary Incontinence During Intercourse: A Review on an Understudied Problem for Women's Sexuality.

Maurizio Serati, et al; 2009. J Sex Med.

Update in Female Hormonal Therapy: What the Urologist Should Know.

Nirit Rosenblum, 2020. Rev Urol.

The Effect of Genital Prolapse on Voiding.

Lauri Romanzi, et al; 1999. J Urol.

Obstetrics and Fecal Incontinence.

Kathleen Chin, et al; 2014. Clin Colon Rectal Surg.

Chapter 5

Imaging Modalities for Pelvic Floor Disorders.

Giulio Aniello Santoro, et al; 2022. Annals of Laparoscopic and Endoscopic Surgery (ALES)

Chapter 6

Seven-year Efficacy and Safety Outcomes of Bulkamid for the Treatment of Stress Urinary Incontinence.

Torsten Brosche, et al; 2021. Neurourol Urodyn.

Chapter 7

Pelvic Organ Prolapse in Women: Choosing a Primary Surgical Procedure.

J Eric Jelovsek, et al; 2020. Lancet.

Chapter 8

Colpocleisis as an Obliterative Surgery for Pelvic Organ Prolapse: Is it still a Viable Option in the Twenty-first Century? Narrative Review.

Magdalena Emilia Grzybowska, et al; 2022. Int Urogynecol J.

Chapter 14

Obstetrics and Gynecology Devices Panel of the Medical Devices Advisory Committee; Notice of Meeting.

2011. Federal Register, The Daily Journal of the United States Government.

Pelvic Organ Prolapse (POP): Surgical Mesh Considerations and Recommendations.

2021. U.S. Food and Drug Administration.

Chapter 17

Epidemiology and Outcome Assessment of Pelvic Organ Prolapse.

Matthew Barber, et al; 2013. Int Urogynecol J.Diagnosed Prevalence of Ehlers-Danlos Syndrome and Hypermobility Spectrum Disorder in Wales, UK: A National Electronic Cohort Study and Case–control Comparison.

Joanne Demmler, et al; 2019. BMJ Open.

Recent Studies of Genetic Dysfunction in Pelvic Organ Prolapse: The Role of Collagen Defects.

Veronica Lim, et al; 2014. Aust N Z J Obstet Gynaecol.

Are Women with Pelvic Organ Prolapse at a Higher Risk of Developing Hernias?

Yakir Segev, et al; 2009. Int Urogynecol J.

Ehlers-Danlos syndrome and Hypermobility Spectrum Disorders in the Context of Childbearing: An International Qualitative Study.

Sally Pezaro, et al; 2020. Midwivery.

Ehlers-danlos Syndrome: It's not your Normal Hoofbeats. Laura Hein, et al; 2019. J Nurse Pract.

Histopathological Evaluation of the Connective Tissue of the Vaginal Fascia and the Uterine Ligaments in Women with and without Pelvic Relaxation. Arif Kökçü, et al; 2002. Arch Gynecol Obstet.

Quality of Life in the Classic and Hypermobility Types of Ehlers-Danlos Syndrome [corrected].

Marco Castori, et al; 2010. Ann Neurol.

Changes in Connective Tissue in Patients with Pelvic Organ Prolapse--A Review of the Current Literature. MH Manon, et al; 2009. Urogynecol J Pelvic Floor Dysfunct.

Urogenital and Pelvic Complications in the Ehlers-Danlos Syndromes and Associated Hypermobility Spectrum Disorders: A Scoping Review.

Elizabeth Gilliam, et al; 2020. Clin Genet.

Gynecologic and Obstetric Implications of the Joint Hypermobility Syndrome (a.k.a. Ehlers-Danlos Syndrome Hypermobility Type) in 82 Italian Patients.

Marco Castori, et al; 2012. Am J Med Genet A.

A Guide for the Issues & Management of Ehlers-Danlos Syndrome Hypermobility Type and The Hypermobility Syndrome. Brad Tinkle, 2009. Left Paw Press.

Prevalence of Urinary and Faecal Incontinence among Female Members of the Hypermobility Syndrome Association (HMSA). Anga Arunkalaivanan, et al; 2009. J Obstet Gynaecol.

Pregnancy and the Ehlers-Danlos Syndrome: A Retrospective Study in a Dutch Population: Ehlers-Danlos Syndrome and Pregnancy.

Jan Lind, et al; 2002. ACTA Obstet Gynecol Scand.

Pelvic Organ Prolapse and Collagen-associated Disorders. Karin Lammers, et al; 2012. Int Urogynecol J.

Genitourinary Prolapse and Joint Hypermobility are Associated with altered Type I and III Collagen Metabolism.

E Knutti, et al; 2011. Arch Gynecol Obstet.

Regulation of Extracellular Matrix Remodeling Associated with Pelvic Organ Prolapse.

Ming-Ping Wu; 2010. J Exp Clin Med.

Chapter 18

Levator Avulsion: Simply Explained.

Sue Croft; 2016. Association for Pelvic Organ Prolapse Support.

Levator Ani Muscle Volume and Architecture in Normal vs. Muscle Damage Patients using 3D Endovaginal Ultrasound: A Pilot Study.

Zara Asif, et al; 2022. Int Urogynecol J.

The Levator Ani Muscle Repair: A Call to Action.

R. Tomashev, et al; 2021. Spring Link.

Chapter 20

Coital Incontinence in Women with Urinary Incontinence: An International Study.

Ester Illiano, et al; 2018. Epub.

INDEX

A

abdominal pain, 19

adenomyosis, 195

B

biofeedback, 46, 76, 77, 96

bioidentical hormone replacement, 60

bladder, 5, 17, 22, 41, 42, 49, 53, 55-58, 63, 71, 75, 89, 97, 136, 143, 147, 155, 167, 170

bridging, 211

C

catheter, 41, 106, 107

childbirth, xvi, 6, 15-17, 22, 41, 43, 53, 64, 72, 75, 135, 168, 187, 188, 198, 206

chronic coughing, 20, 74, 216

coital incontinence, 8, 32, 167, 170, 171, 207

collagen, 19, 64, 66, 70, 96, 144, 147

colpocleisis, 85-87, 89, 176

constipation, xvi, 8, 9, 16, 19, 27, 29-31, 55, 79, 87, 92, 110, 113, 134, 135, 142,

I

IBS, 25, 26, 41, 42, 157, 191, 258

incontinence, xvii, 8, 17, 18, 23, 26-33, 41-43, 48, 52, 55-57, 59, 64, 65, 68, 69, 72-76, 79, 80, 88, 89, 92, 96, 97, 103, 105, 117, 118, 135, 142, 143, 146, 154, 161-165, 167, 169-171, 180, 207, 209, 213, 218

irritable bowel, 25, 35

K

kegel exercises, 37, 53, 72, 150

KY jelly, 110, 212

KY ultra liquid, 109, 212

L

labia, 51, 135, 136

levator ani, 17, 53, 54, 149, 151, 153-158

levator avulsion, 149, 151, 153, 157, 158

M

Marfan syndrome, 19

menopause, 6, 17, 18, 42, 53, 59, 60, 63, 68, 97, 129, 130, 187, 202, 208, 215

mixed urinary incontinence, 37, 39, 106

multiple sclerosis, 21

N

non-surgical treatment options, 45, 46, 92, 105, 217

O

obesity, 16, 20

overactive bladder, 55-57, 65, 71, 75, 89, 167

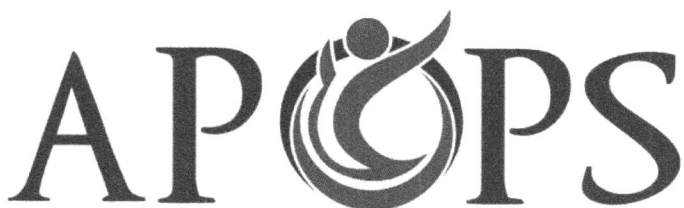

ASSOCIATION FOR PELVIC ORGAN PROLAPSE SUPPORT

ABOUT APOPS

Association for Pelvic Organ Prolapse Support (APOPS) is a USA based 501(c)(3) nonprofit patient advocacy agency with global arms, founded in September 2010 to generate awareness of pelvic organ prolapse (POP), to provide support and guidance to women navigating the physical, emotional, social, sexual, fitness, and employment quality of life impacts of POP, and to bridge the patient, healthcare, industry, research, and academic communities for the betterment of POP understanding and treatment evolution.

MISSION STATEMENT

APOPS mission is to engender pelvic organ prolapse awareness, to listen to and acknowledge patient voice, to destigmatize vaginal health, to encourage and optimize vaginal health empowerment, and to clarify and quantify POP quality of life ramifications.

VISION STATEMENT

APOPS vision is a world in which pelvic organ prolapse awareness and screening are standardized aspects of women's pelvic wellness checks, and vaginal health stigma has been eradicated.

APOPS website is https://www.pelvicorganprolapsesupport.org.

*APOPS website
QR code.*

APOPS GOALS

Immediate Goals:

1. Amplify pelvic organ prolapse awareness.

2. Provide global pelvic organ prolapse guidance and support.

3. Bridge with key stakeholders and organizations to evolve understanding of and evolution in POP treatment.

Long-Term Goals:

1. Inclusion of standardized POP screening in pelvic exams.

2. Accurate statistical data capture.

3. Advancement of diagnostic clinician POP curriculum.

ABOUT THE AUTHOR

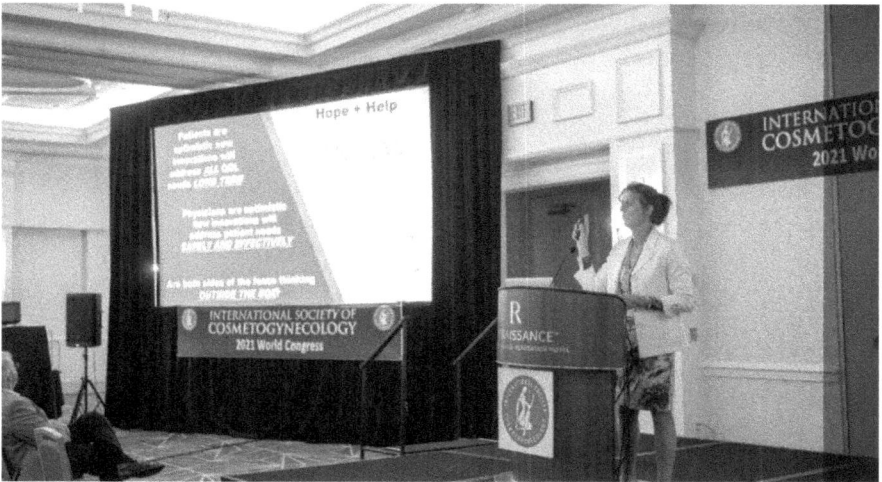

Sherrie Palm presenting at International Society of Cosmetogynecology.

Sherrie Palm carves the global trail to de-stigmatize pelvic organ prolapse (POP), a common women's health condition impacting an estimated 50% of women, as she educates and inspires to facilitate evolution of women's health directives.

Sherrie Palm is the Founder/CEO of APOPS, Association for Pelvic Organ Prolapse Support, author of *The Biggest Secret in Women's Health: Stigma, Indifference, Outrage, and Optimism*, author of three editions of the award-winning book *Pelvic Organ Prolapse: The Silent Epidemic*, a pelvic organ prolapse patient advocate, vaginal and intimate health activist, internationally recognized speaker, POP key opinion leader, and prolific writer regarding POP physical, emotional, social, sexual, fitness, and employment quality of life impacts.

Sherrie has presented speeches nationally and internationally to physician, research, academic, corporate, government policy, and patient audiences since 2011. Her points of focus are increasing awareness of the next significant evolution in women's health awareness, screening, practice, and policy, advancing women's vaginal and intimate health empowerment, developing POP patient guidance and support structures, and bridge-building within patient and professional sectors toward the advancement of women's pelvic health and POP best practice.

Recognizing a need to shift the global view of the remaining stigmatized aspects of women's health, Sherrie Palm takes steps to pioneer change. Cognizant of the diverse and sensitive needs of her audience, Sherrie delicately places all the cards on the table to disclose aspects of vaginal health and intimate wellness rarely effectively discussed. Sherrie's capacity to respectfully and compassionately answer all questions posed during speaking engagements endears her to the audience.

Submit queries related to APOPS or Ms. Palm's presentation availability via:

https://www.pelvicorganprolapsesupport.org/contact

Sign up for APOPS news at:

https://www.tinyurl.com/APOPSnews

PLEASE MAKE A DONATION TO ASSIST APOPS EFFORTS TO SUPPORT WOMEN WITH POP

APOPS is a federally designated 501(c)(3) nonprofit organization. If the information in this book has helped you on your journey to find answers for or educate patients with POP, please consider assisting our efforts to build tools to guide women experiencing pelvic organ prolapse by making a donation.

Google **APOPS + DONATE** or click on the link or QR code below.

https://www.pelvicorganprolapsesupport.org/make-a-donation

Letter from APOPS Founder, September 8, 2010

From the beginning of this journey, I knew I wanted to connect with women on a deeper level about the impact POP has on our lives. Those of us who have already been diagnosed and treated for POP understand the distress women newly diagnosed are going through. It can be frustrating to dissect the information available. Is the data we have access to accurate? Which information applies to us personally? Are nonsurgical treatments or surgery the best path? It takes a bit of time to figure out the right course to take.

My vision for APOPS is simple - women who are a bit further down the path of POP awareness connecting with women who are newly diagnosed. Together we will find the information that will assist our paths. Together we will guide, support, and nurture each other. Together we will shift the awareness curve by passing the information we gain on to the younger generation.

I have no doubt that with the strength and determination women bring to the table, we will change the mindset of the world at large, transforming pelvic organ prolapse, the insufficiently acknowledged women's health condition, to a widely recognized health disorder that is routinely screened for to enable early diagnosis and treatment for continuing quality of life.

My continuing gratitude to you all!

· · · ● · ● · ● · · ·

"For a health condition to remain shrouded in silence because of embarrassment at this point in history, after all we have achieved as women, is unacceptable."

Sherrie Palm

www.ingramcontent.com/pod-product-compliance
Lightning Source LLC
Chambersburg PA
CBHW041255040426
42334CB00028BA/3024